RAPID NURSING INTERVENTIONS:

$\mathscr{P}$ediatric

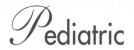

Delmar Publishers' Online Services

To access Delmar on the World Wide Web, point your browser to:
    http://www.delmar.com/delmar.html

To access through Gopher:
    gopher://gopher.delmar.com

(Delmar Online is part of "thomson.com," an Internet site with information on more than 30 publishers of the International Thomson Publishing organization.)

For more information on our products and services:
    email: info@delmar.com or call 800-347-7707

RAPID NURSING INTERVENTIONS:

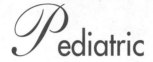

$\mathscr{P}$ediatric

▽   ▽   ▽   ▽   ▽   ▽   ▽

Monika E. Bauman, RN, BSN, CEN
Senior Partner
Pediatric Emergency Department
University of Maryland Medical System
Baltimore

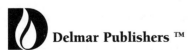 **Delmar Publishers ™**

I⟨T⟩P™ An International Thomson Publishing Company

Albany • Bonn • Boston • Cincinnati • Detroit • London • Madrid
Melbourne • Mexico City • New York • Pacific Grove • Paris • San Francisco
Singapore • Tokyo • Toronto • Washington

$\mathscr{S}$TAFF

▼ **Team Leader:**
DIANE McOSCAR

▼ **Sponsoring Editors:**
▼ PATRICIA CASEY
▼ BILL BURGOWER

▼ **Developed for Delmar Publishers Inc by:**
▼ JENNINGS & KEEFE Media Development, Corte Madera, CA

▼ **Concept, Editorial, and Design Management:**
▼ THE WILLIAMS COMPANY, LTD., Collegeville, PA

▼ **Project Coordinator:**
▼ KATHLEEN LUCZAK

▼ **Editorial Administrator:**
▼ GABRIEL DAVIS

▼ **Production Editor:**
▼ BARBARA HODGSON

▼ **Senior Book Editor:**
▼ TERRI A. GREENBERG

▼ **Book Editor:**
▼ JOANN NASH

Text Design:
KM DESIGN GROUP

For information, address:
Delmar Publishers
3 Columbia Circle
Box 15015
Albany, NY 12212-5015

International Thomson Publishing Europe
Berkshire House 168-173
High Holborn
London, WC1V7AA
England

Thomas Nelson Australia
102 Dodds Street
South Melbourne, 3205
Victoria, Australia

Nelson Canada
1120 Birchmount Road
Scarborough, Ontario
Canada M1K 5G4

International Thomson Editores
Campos Eliseos 385, Piso 7
Col Polanco
11560 Mexico D F Mexico

International Thomson Publishing GmbH
Königswinterer Strasse 418
53227 Bonn
Germany

International Thomson Publishing Asia
221 Henderson Road
#05-10 Henderson Building
Singapore 0315

International Thomson Publishing Japan
Hirakawacho Kyowa Building, 3F
2-2-1 Hirakawacho
Chiyoda-ku, Tokyo 102
Japan

Printed in the United States of America

Published simultaneously in Canada by Nelson Canada, a division of The Thomson Corporation.

1 2 3 4 5 6 7 8 9 10 XXX 00 99 98 97 96 95

Library of Congress Cataloging-in-Publication Data
Bauman, Monika E., 1968-
        Rapid nursing interventions: pediatric/Monika E. Bauman
        p.   cm. — (Rapid nursing interventions)
        Includes bibliographical references and index.
        ISBN 0-8273-7097-0
        1. Pediatric nursing—Handbooks, manuals, etc. I. Title.
        II. Series.
        [DNLM: 1. Pediatric Nursing—methods—handbooks.
        2. Nursing Process—handbooks. WY 49 B347r 1996]
        RJ245.B38 1996
        610.73'62—dc20
        DNLM/DLC
        for Library of Congress   95-20855
                                                        CIP

TITLES IN THIS SERIES:

INSTANT NURSING ASSESSMENT:

▲ Cardiovascular

▲ Respiratory

▲ Neurologic

▲ Women's Health

▲ Gerontologic

▲ Mental Health

▲ Pediatric

RAPID NURSING INTERVENTIONS:

▲ Cardiovascular

▲ Respiratory

▲ Neurologic

▲ Women's Health

▲ Gerontologic

▲ Mental Health

▲ Pediatric

Suzanne K. Marnocha, RN, MSN, CCRN
Assistant Professor, College of Nursing
University of Wisconsin
Oshkosh, Wisconsin

Linda Moody, RN, FAAN, Ph.D.
Professor, Director of Research and Chair,
Gerontology Nursing
College of Nursing
University of South Florida
Tampa, Florida

Patricia A. O'Neill, RN, CCRN, MSN
Instructor, DeAnza College School of Nursing
Cupertino, California

Virgil Parsons, RN, DNSc, Ph.D.
Professor, School of Nursing
San Jose State University
San Jose, California

Elaine Rooney, MSN
Assistant Professor of Nursing, Nursing Department
University of Pittsburgh
Bradford, Pennsylvania

Barbara Shafner, RN, Ph.D.
Associate Professor, Department of Nursing
Otterbein College
Westerville, Ohio

Elaine Souder, RN, Ph.D.
Associate Professor, College of Nursing
University of Arkansas for Medical Sciences
Little Rock, Arkansas

Mary Tittle, RN, Ph.D.
Associate Professor, College of Nursing
University of South Florida
Tampa, Florida

Peggy L. Wros, RN, Ph.D.
Assistant Professor of Nursing
Linfield College School of Nursing
Portland, Oregon

CONTENTS

Section I. Symptoms and Interventions Review

CHAPTER 1.   SYMPTOMS AND FOCUSED ASSESSMENT   1

CHAPTER 2.   NURSING INTERVENTIONS   6

Section II. Health Maintenance

CHAPTER 3.   HEALTH HISTORY   13

CHAPTER 4.   PHYSICAL ASSESSMENT   22

Section III. Systemic Review

CHAPTER 5.   HEAD AND NECK   37

CHAPTER 6.   RESPIRATORY SYSTEM   51

CHAPTER 7.   CARDIOVASCULAR SYSTEM   64

CHAPTER 8.   GASTROINTESTINAL SYSTEM   83

CHAPTER 9.   REPRODUCTIVE SYSTEM   95

CHAPTER 10. RENAL AND URINARY SYSTEM   113

CHAPTER 11. MUSCULOSKELETAL SYSTEM   122

CHAPTER 12. NEUROLOGIC SYSTEM   137

CHAPTER 13. SKIN AND LYMPH SYSTEM   147

Section IV. Common Problems

CHAPTER 14. FEVER   159

CHAPTER 15. CHILDHOOD INFECTIONS   168

CHAPTER 16. POISONING AND INGESTIONS   182

CHAPTER 17. TRAUMA   188

CHAPTER 18. SHOCK   196

Appendix

Index

NOTICE TO THE READER

The publisher, editors, advisors, and reviewers do not warrant or guarantee any of the products described herein nor have they performed any independent analysis in connection with any of the product information contained herein. The publisher, editors, advisors, and reviewers do not assume, and each expressly disclaims, any obligation to obtain and include information other than that provided to them by the manufacturer.

The reader is expressly warned to consider and adopt all safety precautions that might be indicated by the activities described herein and to avoid all potential hazards. By following the instructions contained herein, the reader willingly assumes all risks in connection with such instructions.

The publisher, editors, advisors, and reviewers make no representations or warranties of any kind, including but not limited to the warranties of fitness for particular purpose or merchantability, nor are any such representations implied with respect to the material set forth herein, and the publisher, editors, advisors, and reviewers take no responsibility with respect to such material. The publisher, editors, advisors, and reviewers shall not be liable for any special, consequential, or exemplary damages resulting, in whole or in part, from readers' use of, or reliance upon, this material.

A conscientious effort has been made to ensure that the drug information and recommended dosages in this book are accurate and in accord with accepted standards at the time of publication. However, pharmacology is a rapidly changing science, so readers are advised, before administering any drug, to check the package insert provided by the manufacturer for the recommended dose, for contraindications for administration, and for added warnings and precautions. This recommendation is especially important for new, infrequently used, or highly toxic drugs.

CPR standards are subject to frequent change due to ongoing research. The American Heart Association can verify changing CPR standards when applicable. Recommended Schedules for Immunization are also subject to frequent change. The American Academy of Pediatrics, Committee on Infectious Diseases can verify changing recommendations.

FOREWORD

As quality and cost effectiveness continue to drive rapid change within the health-care system, you must respond quickly and sure-ly—whether you are a student, novice, or expert. This Rapid Nursing Interventions series—and its companion Instant Nursing Assessment series—will help you do that by providing a great deal of nursing information in short, easy-to-read columns, charts and boxes. This quick, convenient presentation will support you as you practice your science and art and apply the nursing process. I hope you'll come to look on these books as providing "an experi-enced nurse in your pocket."

The Rapid Nursing Interventions series is a handy source for step-by-step nursing actions to meet the fast-paced challenges of today's nursing profession. The Instant Nursing Assessment series offers immediate, relevant clinical information on the most important aspects of patient assessment. These books contain several helpful special features, including nurse alerts to warn you quickly about critical assessment findings, nursing diagnoses, charts that include interventions and rationales, along with collaborative management to help you work with your health-care colleagues, patient teach-ing tips, and the latest nursing research findings.

Each title in the Rapid Nursing Interventions series begins with a quick review of symptoms and focused assessment followed by the components of nursing intervention. From there, each book expands to cover the essential nursing interventions and ratio-nales, collaborative management, outcomes, and evaluation crite-ria for important diagnoses covered in that title.

Both medical and nursing diagnoses are included to help you adapt to emerging critical pathways, care mapping, and decision trees. All these new guidelines help decrease length-of-stay and increase quality of care—all current health-care imperatives.

I'm confident that each small but powerful volume will prove indispensable in your nursing practice. Each book is formatted to help you quickly connect your assessment findings with the patient's pathophysiology—a cognitive connection that will further help you plan nursing interventions, both independent and collab-orative, to care for your patients skillfully and completely. With the help and guidance provided by the books in this series, you will be able to thrive—and survive—in these changing times.

— Helene K. Nawrocki, RN, MSN, CNA
Executive Vice President
The Center for Nursing Excellence
Newtown, Pennsylvania
Adjunct Faculty, La Salle University
Philadelphia, Pennsylvania

SECTION I. SYMPTOMS AND INTERVENTIONS REVIEW

Chapter 1. Symptoms and Focused Assessment

▽   ▽   ▽   ▽   ▽   ▽   ▽

Introduction

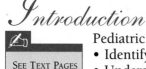

SEE TEXT PAGES

Pediatric physical assessment involves the following:
- Identifying signs and symptoms
- Understanding the health care implications of the physiologic aspects of the pediatric patient
- Understanding the child's developmental level and the effects of the illness or injury on the child at that stage of development
- Communicating effectively with the child and the child's family
- Listening to the parents or primary caregivers because they know the child best

In the care of all children, it is essential to recognize potentially life-threatening problems that require intervention.

Evaluating children is more difficult than evaluating adults for a number of reasons. Symptoms, such as fever, may be less specific in children. Communication is more difficult because a third party—the parent or guardian—is frequently the major source of most of the history.

Each child occupies a special position in the family; the family as a whole is usually involved in the care of each child. Support must be provided to the sick or injured child while undue disruption to normal family routine is avoided. Illness, injury, and hospitalization may cause a crisis for the child and family. The family's ability to cope with illness is influenced by the event, the support systems available to them, and their past experiences in coping with stressful situations. Many caregivers blame themselves for a child's illness or accident. Some even try to explain an illness or accident as a "punishment" or as some manifestation of "God's will."

How the family responds to the child's illness or injury is also influenced by environmental and personal resource networks. The environmental resources include initial encounters with health care staff and the attitudes and interventions they offer. Relatives and friends are among the personal resources available to the family.

The nurse is in a position to assess the family structure and dynamics and the important implications they have for the child's well-care, illness, and recovery. The traditional family structure is becoming less common because many children are being raised by single parents or grandparents or are members of blended families with stepparents and stepsiblings.

Assessment and intervention for the pediatric patient present unique challenges. Both management and the plan of care must be communicated to the whole family. Family-centered emotional, psychological, and educational support must be given to the family as well as to the ill or injured child.

A child's response to illness and injury depends on the child's developmental stage. Children may not appear outwardly symptomatic, even when their condition is life-threatening, because they can compensate for impaired functioning for longer periods than adults. Symptoms may be subtle; once a child's condition deteriorates, interventions must be rapid. The child's vital signs may be difficult to assess and the approach must be geared to developmental level and the right equipment.

Observation, examination, and communication with the child and parents are the major components of pediatric assessment.

Observation

Begin the assessment with a general observation of the child's appearance. Does the child look sick? Is the child clean and well groomed? Is the child reacting appropriately in the medical setting? How does the child interact with the family? Do the parents or caregivers seem concerned, or indifferent?

Observe for signs and symptoms of respiratory distress. Does the child's color appear normal? Is the child's skin pale, blotchy, or cyanotic? Observe the nail beds and mucous membranes for signs of cyanosis. Is the child using accessory muscles in the neck or chest? Is there nasal flaring or retractions? Is the child's breathing noisy? A barking cough or crowing respirations may point to upper airway obstruction. Wheezing indicates lower airway obstruction.

Examination

Primary

The initial examination of the child includes assessment of the airway, breathing, and circulation—the ABCs—as well as a brief neurologic assessment and vital signs evaluation.

Airway, Breathing, and Circulation

Assessment begins by checking the ABCs:
- Airway for patency and evidence of impairment
- Breathing for signs of respiratory insufficiency or distress
- Circulation for signs of impairment

Neurologic Examination

A brief neurologic examination should be included in the primary assessment of all patients. This examination should include the child's level of consciousness and orientation. Is the child awake, alert, and playful, or lethargic and listless? A more detailed examination may be recommended based on initial findings. For example, if a child who presents with a head injury is lethargic, a more in-depth neurologic assessment is necessary.

Vital Signs

Obtain vital signs, including temperature, pulse rate, respiratory rate, blood pressure, and weight. Be alert to the fact that normal vital signs—specifically blood pressure—may give a false sense of security. For example, children in the early stage of shock have a normal blood pressure reading because of their ability to compensate for diminished function.

NURSE ALERT:
A dropping blood pressure is a serious sign that needs immediate intervention.

Is the child's weight within normal range? Weight should be obtained in kilograms. It is an important factor in calculating medication doses and fluid administration, assessing for degree of dehydration, and comparing growth and development with the normal growth and development for a specific age-group. A child's birth weight normally doubles by 5 to 6 months of age and triples by 1 year of age.

Secondary

The secondary assessment may be conducted in a head-to-toe manner, as a systems review, or as a problem-focused assessment. It includes an in-depth assessment for injury or illness and specific assessment based on the primary complaint.

In the secondary assessment, the child is undressed for a thorough physical examination. At this time, a more detailed and comprehensive assessment is performed. Refer to Chapter 4, which covers the head-to-toe examination in more detail. Check for signs of serious illness or injury. Use your "sixth sense" in this phase of the assessment to add your subjective feeling or intuition regarding the child's condition to the objective data obtained.

In emergency situations, the primary assessment may include appropriate interventions before secondary assessment is begun. For example, the child may require oxygen and ventilatory support before a head-to-toe examination is begun.

Communication

Communication must be clear and focused on reducing fear and anxiety. Open lines of communication are needed to provide comfort to the child, parents, and siblings as well as to other members of the child's support network throughout all procedures. Enhanced communication channels help to reduce psychological trauma and ensure cooperation with all parties.

Communicate with the child based on what is appropriate for his or her age and developmental level. Direct interaction with the child enhances both the assessment procedure and the success of interventions.

Communicate with the parents or other caregivers in an understanding, empathetic manner. Do not be judgmental even if a complaint or question seems trivial; everyone is concerned with the child's health and well-being. Listen to the caregiver; this person may intuitively know that the child is not well.

TRANSCULTURAL CONSIDERATIONS
The family who is of a culture different from your own presents a unique challenge. Assess the effectiveness of your communication with the family, and consult appropriate resources to serve as a translator when needed. Be sure to clarify any cultural issues you think might be raised by your treatment of the child with the parents or caregivers.

Chapter 2. Nursing Interventions

▽   ▽   ▽   ▽   ▽   ▽   ▽

Introduction

SEE TEXT PAGES

Several critical aspects lead to efficient and effective nursing interventions with pediatric patients. A rapport must be established with both the child and the parents or caregivers. Remember that management of the pediatric patient should be directed toward the entire family—primary caregivers, siblings, and other significant members of the child's support network as well as the child. A quiet, nondisruptive area is needed for the examination, and appropriate equipment must be ready for the assessment.

Communication

Keep channels of communication open, beginning with the assessment and continuing throughout any interventions. Providing emotional and psychological support to the child and caregivers is an important component of the care of a sick or injured child. The effectiveness of your interventions to support both the child and the family depends on certain factors, such as the child's age, developmental level, personality, fears, coping mechanisms, and physical condition.

Interventions to ease caregiver stress should reduce environmental factors as well as those factors associated with the health care situation or family background. Acknowledge concerns about being absent from a job or caring for other children; assess perceptions of health, attitudes, support systems, and financial resources. Offer referrals or assistance as needed.

After the initial greeting of family and child, approach the child gently and explain what you are going to do before you do it. Convey a patient, calm, supportive, nonjudgmental attitude toward everyone concerned. Be warm and respectful toward the patient and family. This shows your friendliness and consideration as well as your respect for the patient's and family's worth and individuality.

Appropriate information, guidance, support, and resources help the family care for the child. By establishing a trusting relationship with family members, you can do much to ease any anxiety they may have about the child's health.

Begin by giving specific information about the child's condition and treatment. Explain the nature of the child's physical status, injury, or illness. Discuss the physiologic and behavioral changes that can be expected during the course of any illness or injury.

Provide frequent reports about the child's progress. Adequately explain all procedures, operations, or therapies related to the child's health and well-being. Be frank and consistent in your explanations, making sure that all the child's caregivers provide the same consistent information.

Repeat and clarify information as often as seems necessary. Frequently caregivers need this repetition and clarification about the child's health, particularly if the child is very ill or has been injured. Much of the information given during the early stages of an emergency is lost because initial shock and disbelief limit the caregivers' ability to listen and comprehend and decrease accurate perception.

Encourage caregivers to be present and assist in the child's care. They can continue to serve in an important role even in the hospital setting by participating in the child's care. Aid them in staying calm and cooperative, which helps lessen the child's anxiety. Providing direct care to the child seems to promote better coping with anxiety and possible guilt feelings about the child's illness or injury.

Help define the caregivers' role and tell them just what they can do for the child. Their role in the health care setting should be an extension of the one they perform in the home. Support them and compliment them for their efforts. This fosters support of the child by allowing them to function in a familiar, comfortable manner. Their roles as primary providers of comfort, warmth, nourishment, and rest to their child should continue. Encourage caregivers to touch the child to calm and divert him or her. Allow them to hold the child, to provide explanations, to reassure, and to communicate directly with the child.

Parents or caregivers can be valuable allies and should be allowed to remain with the child whenever possible. Not only does this help obtain the child's cooperation, but it also supports the family unit. In addition, caregivers who are close at hand can provide important information that may have an impact on the child's care.

Most parents or caregivers know their child better than anyone else. They usually can explain procedures in a way the child will understand, and they know how to help the child cope with the circumstances. Participating in the child's care makes them feel needed and useful and that the child is still theirs.

Attend to the caregivers' and siblings' needs as well. Other family members may be upset or frightened. Give them the opportunity to express their feelings, concerns, fears, and frustrations; allow them private moments as well. Single parents may have special requirements because they may feel alone and frightened. Single as well as dual-caregiver families may be faced with issues related to child care of other siblings and the inability to take time off from work. Give permission for them to take a break. Encourage the parents and other caregivers to maintain relationships with one another, with their other children, and with other relatives and friends. Provide referrals to sources of financial aid and counseling.

Explore the role of religion in the family's life. Offer referrals to clergy as appropriate.

Ask about other children in the family and any others who are important in the lives of the child and caregivers. Allow siblings to be present if their presence will benefit the sick child. Explain the illness or injury to siblings, who sometimes resent the disruptions in their lives caused by a brother's or sister's illness or injury. In cases of an emergency illness or injury, the family naturally focuses on the sick child. This focus tends to create disequilibrium within the family that intensifies sibling rivalries and decreases the benefit of sibling-patient relationships. By explaining the situation to siblings, you help decrease their feelings of loneliness and isolation when the family's attention is on the sick or injured child.

Vital Signs

Vital signs in the pediatric patient may vary from normal for a number of reasons. The major concern is to watch for signs that the child may be critically ill or approaching a crisis situation and may need immediate intervention.

For example, distinguish between the child with increased heart and respiratory rates resulting from shock or other emergent illness and the child whose increased rates are due to pain, crying, anxiety, or physical exertion. Immediate intervention may be necessary in the child with acute distress, whereas you can progress to a general or focused examination in the child who does not seem seriously ill.

Respirations

A child with symptoms of severe respiratory distress (ineffective or inadequate respiration) requires immediate interventions, which may include securing and clearing the airway, assisting ventilation with 100% oxygen, and, ultimately, instituting endotracheal intubation and mechanical ventilation. Refer to the American Heart Association and American Academy of Pediatrics guidelines for pediatric advanced life support. Immediate intervention of supplemental oxygen administered by face mask, nasal cannula, or the "blow by" technique may be sufficient.

The child who is in respiratory distress may need other interventions, including the following:
• To be maintained in a position of comfort
• To be held by the parent or caregiver
• To be assessed by a physician as soon as possible
• To be monitored for other signs of increasing distress and indications of impending respiratory failure

Upper airway problems produce primarily ventilatory abnormalities related to partial or absolute obstruction. Lower airway disorders may impair ventilation perfusion. Because airway problems may stem from a variety of conditions, interventions beyond those described above focus on the cause of respiratory distress.

NURSE ALERT:
Children may progress rapidly to respiratory failure and arrest and, subsequently, to cardiac arrest. Respiratory distress must be treated expediently.

Pulse

Abnormal pulse rates may be described as too fast (the tachyarrhythmias) or too slow (the bradyarrhythmias).

A heart rate that is rapid may not require immediate treatment other than eliminating the cause—for example, by administering acetaminophen for fever. When the heart rate becomes so rapid that there are clinical signs of compromised perfusion (decreased level of consciousness), interventions for basic and advanced life support should be implemented. Interventions depend on the type of rhythm that is present. Regardless of the rhythm, nursing interventions are aimed at initiating ECG monitoring, establishing I.V. access, and prompting immediate physician assessment.

A heart rate that is too slow (bradycardia) in the pediatric patient is most commonly caused by hypoxia resulting from inadequate ventilation. Interventions are aimed at ensuring an adequate airway and ventilation. Other conditions that may cause bradycardia include drug ingestion, heart block, and increased intracranial pressure. Interventions in these instances focus on treatment of the cause, such as treating drug toxicity, initiating cardiac pacing, relieving increased intracranial pressure, and administering medications, such as atropine.

Blood Pressure

Elevated blood pressure in children may be caused by anxiety or by other pathology, such as renal failure. Intervention in this situation is aimed at eliminating the cause of anxiety and administering hypertensives, as ordered.

Decreased blood pressure (hypotension) in children is a more common and serious finding and may result from such conditions as pump failure (congestive heart failure), loss of significant circulating volume (hypovolemia), and peripheral vasodilation (septic shock). Interventions must be immediate, aggressive, and aimed at treating the cause. Interventions may include volume replacement, vasopressors, and antibiotics, as indicated. In all these circumstances, I.V. access is initiated with close monitoring of blood pressure trends, pulse rate, and patient's response to therapy. I.V. access is more difficult in the pediatric patient, particularly one who is hypovolemic. Determine fluid replacement based on both the child's estimated volume loss and the child's weight in kilograms. (A child has about 80 mL of blood volume per kilogram of weight.)

NURSE ALERT:
To obtain accurate blood pressure measurements, the proper size equipment must be available. A cuff that is too large will give a low reading, and a cuff that is too small will give a high reading.

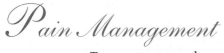

Pain Management

To manage procedure-related pain, give the child and his or her family adequate and developmentally appropriate information about the procedure. Make sure the environment is comfortable and that there is privacy, good lighting, and no distracting noise. Explain expected roles to parents and caregivers, and allow them to be with the child throughout the procedure. When possible, combine pharmacologic and nonpharmacologic choices. Make sure the child has received maximal treatment for pain and anxiety related to the first procedure to minimize anticipatory anxiety before a procedure is repeated.

NURSE ALERT:
When a local or systemic analgesic is not used, be alert to the child who does not respond to painful procedures. This is the sign of a very ill child!

Pharmacologic collaborative interventions include the use of analgesics or local anesthetics, which are used for the management of painful procedures. Anxiolytics and sedatives specifically reduce associated anxiety. If these medications are used alone, behavioral responses are blocked, but pain is not relieved. Systemic analgesics can be used alone or with anxiolytics or sedatives. Skilled supervision and appropriate monitoring are essential when systemic analgesics and sedatives are given.

Other considerations in the use of pharmacologic agents include the following:
• Both injected and topical local anesthetics reduce pain sensation. I.V., I.M., and oral opioids produce analgesia. When given I.V., they may be titrated to the desired effect.

- Oral or I.V. benzodiazepines produce anxiolysis and sedation but not analgesia. I.V. benzodiazepines should be given in increments and titrated to effect.
- Oral or I.V. barbiturates offer sedation but no analgesic effect.
- Other agents, such as nitrous oxide and ketamine, may be used when skilled personnel and appropriate monitoring are available.
- General anesthetics may be appropriate at times.

Nonpharmacologic strategies for less painful procedures, such as venipuncture, can be used alone or as adjuncts to pharmacologic strategies for more painful procedures. They include the following:
- Sensorimotor strategies, such as pacifiers, swaddling, holding, and rocking, for infants
- Cognitive behavioral strategies, such as hypnosis, relaxation, distraction, preparatory information, positive reinforcement, and music, art, and play therapy—all of which can be rehearsed before the procedure
- Child participation strategies that involve the child in age-appropriate decisions about the procedure and aspects of the way it is conducted
- Physical strategies, such as applying heat or cold, massage, exercise, rest, and immobilization
- Nonpharmacologic strategies for older children and adolescents undergoing procedures that are not excessively painful

Suggested Readings

Brantley, D. K. "Communicating with Children: Age-Related Techniques." In *Comprehensive Child and Family Nursing Skills,* edited by D. Smith, 48–53. St. Louis: Mosby-Year Book, 1991.

Herdon, T. R. "Cultural Factors Play a Role in Pediatric Assessment." *Florida Nurse* 38 (February 1990): 11.

Hoekelman, R. "The Physical Examination of Infants and Children." In *A Guide to Physical Examination and History Taking,* edited by Barbara Bates, 561–633. Philadelphia: J. B. Lippincott, 1991.

SECTION II. HEALTH MAINTENANCE

Chapter 3. Health History

▽   ▽   ▽   ▽   ▽   ▽   ▽

Introduction

SEE TEXT PAGES

The child's health history is vital to assessment, especially in emergency situations. The history contains subjective facts about the child and can aid in determining immediate problems and focusing on interventions.

Children are generally healthy and present without histories of chronic conditions or numerous allergies and medications, which usually makes their histories easier to take and more brief. On the other hand, young children and infants cannot speak for themselves, and you must rely on information provided by the parents or other caregivers. Although the caregivers know their child best, you should note your impression of them as a reliable source of information and the level of concern they show about the child's well-being.

Depending on the child's age and developmental stage, ask both the child and the caregiver to describe the child's current condition. Ask what each thinks may have caused any presenting problem and whether either one has any questions or concerns.

To remember the key components of taking a history, use the mnemonic AMPLE:
• Allergies
• Medications
• Past medical history
• Last meal
• Events related to illness or injury

Observe and listen attentively to the child and caregivers while taking a history. Give special consideration to their level of understanding. Match vocabulary and phrase questions to that level. Consider using both verbal and nonverbal aids to communicate. Remember that the ability to communicate and use language varies with age and that a word may have a different meaning based on a child's background and cognitive level.

Always make direct eye contact and listen attentively during responses. Consider the child's developmental level and attention span, and adjust your approach accordingly. Interact with the child first to show that he or she is the primary subject of the history-taking phase of the assessment. If the child is unwilling or unable to respond to the questioning, speak directly with the caregivers.

Use positive reinforcement as the history taking proceeds. Compliment the child. Show empathy by an occasional nod of your head or by saying, "I see." "I understand." "Go on." "Anything else?" and so forth. Do not hinder communication by showing nonverbal distress over an answer or by offering advice during history taking.

Use direct, open-ended, and leading questions. A direct question is quick and useful in getting specific facts, such as name, age, and date of birth. Open-ended questions permit greater freedom for a reply to certain questions. Leading questions are preferred in certain other situations but must be used carefully to avoid getting a biased answer. Such an answer may provide false information because the patient or caregiver is trying to please you by giving the "right" answer.

Document information about the person providing the details of the health history, including the following:
• Reliability
• The identity of the person providing the information: child, parent, or other
• Willingness to communicate
• Special circumstances, such as use of an interpreter or conflicting answers

CHILD'S HEALTH HISTORY

SUBJECT AREA	DESCRIPTION
Demographic	• Name • Age • Date of birth • Gender • Race • Parents' name • Address

CHILD'S HEALTH HISTORY (CONTINUED)

SUBJECT AREA	DESCRIPTION
Demographic (continued)	• Telephone number • Occupation • Insurance • Name of informant • Relationship to patient (mother, father, grandparent, baby-sitter, neighbor)
Chief complaint	Brief account of the problem or reason medical attention has been sought
Present illness	Chronological history surrounding the illness or injury, including: • Influencing factors • Duration • History of symptoms • Related symptoms • Limitations to activity or lifestyle • Onset • Location • Intensity • Degree of pain or discomfort • Actions taken to relieve symptoms
Immunization status	Record of immunization: • What • When • Where • Any adverse reactions
Past medical history	• Past illnesses • Accidents • Injuries • Operations and hospitalizations • Allergies • Current medications (prescribed and unprescribed) • Primary health care source

CHILD'S HEALTH HISTORY (CONTINUED)

SUBJECT AREA	DESCRIPTION
Prenatal and neonatal history	• Length of gestation • Maternal health • Complications • Duration and complications of labor • Birth weight • Need for resuscitation, if any • Length of hospital stay in neonatal intensive care • Need for mechanical ventilation • Duration of mechanical ventilation
Developmental history	Age-related achievements and developmental milestones: • Smiling • Holding head steady • Rolling over • Sitting alone • Crawling, walking • Babbling • Talking • Vocabulary and sentence structure • Riding bicycle • Feeding self • Weaning • Toilet training • Writing, coloring • Tying shoes • Using scissors • Tolerating strangers and separation
Nutritional history	• Bottle- or breast-fed infant • Early feeding difficulties • Vitamin intake • Fluoridation of water • Age of solid food introduction • Frequency of meals • Dietary intake • Food likes and dislikes

CHILD'S HEALTH HISTORY (CONTINUED)

SUBJECT AREA	DESCRIPTION
Family history	• Parental age • Parental health • Marital status • Health of siblings and immediate relatives • Cause of death in close relatives • Family illnesses and conditions
Personality history	• Child's relationship with parents, siblings, and peers • Affect and mood • Disposition (shy, outgoing, aggressive, assertive, extrovert, introvert, talkative, calm, tense, anxious, hyperactive)
Social history	• Income • Home size and number of rooms • Sleeping facilities • Heating, sewage, and water facilities • Education and occupation of parents • Religious affiliation • Racial or ethnic background
Review of systems	• Child's state of health • Recent weight gain or loss • Fatigue • Exercise tolerance Head: • Size • Shape • Fontanelles (open or closed) • Suture lines • Headaches • Dizziness Eyes: • Visual acuity • Visual problems • Redness • Drainage

CHILD'S HEALTH HISTORY (CONTINUED)

SUBJECT AREA	DESCRIPTION
Review of systems (continued)	Eyes: (continued) • Tearing • Unusual movements • Cataracts • Photophobia • Strabismus • Infections • Diplopia or myopia • Glasses or contact lenses Nose: • Stuffiness • Congestion • Drainage • Epistaxis • Postnasal drip • Frequent colds • Smelling ability Mouth: • Teeth: number and condition • Toothaches • Lesions • Ulcers • Mouth breathing • Bleeding gums • Odor • Palate condition Throat: • Soreness • Tonsils • Difficulty swallowing • Hoarseness Ears: • Infections • Drainage • Exudate • Hearing acuity • Earaches • Ringing

CHILD'S HEALTH HISTORY (*CONTINUED*)

SUBJECT AREA	DESCRIPTION
Review of systems (*continued*)	Neck: • Stiffness • Pain • Masses • Enlarged nodes • Tenderness • Movement • Thyroid enlargement Chest: • Breast enlargement • Discharge • Masses • Pain • Self-examination Respiratory: • Dyspnea • Cyanosis • Wheezing • Stridor • Cough • Shortness of breath • Sputum • Hemoptysis Integument: • Color • Rashes • Bruises • Petechiae • Pruritus • Hair loss • Acne • Dryness • Texture Cardiovascular: • Exercise intolerance • Murmurs • Syncope • Anemia

CHILD'S HEALTH HISTORY (CONTINUED)

SUBJECT AREA	DESCRIPTION
Review of systems (continued)	Neurologic: • Seizures • Unsteadiness • Ataxia • Frequent falls • Loss of consciousness • Nervousness • Tremors or twitches • Vertigo • Loss of sensation • Memory loss Gastrointestinal: • Appetite • Anorexia • Feeding problems • Nausea and vomiting • Belching and flatulence • Diarrhea or constipation • Encopresis • Abdominal pain • Jaundice • Anal fissures Genitourinary: • Dysuria or enuresis • Frequency • Urgency or hesitancy • Dribbling • Urinary tract infection • Hematuria • Nocturia • Polyuria • Urine odor • Vaginal or penile discharge • Menses • Sexually transmitted disease Musculoskeletal: • Fractures • Joint swelling or stiffness • Movement limitations • Edema

CHILD'S HEALTH HISTORY *(CONTINUED)*

SUBJECT AREA	DESCRIPTION
Review of systems *(continued)*	Musculoskeletal: *(continued)* • Pain • Deformity • Muscle cramps or spasms • Weakness • Clumsiness • Unusual movements • Sensation or memory loss

Chapter 4. Physical Assessment

▽ ▽ ▽ ▽ ▽ ▽ ▽

Introduction

SEE TEXT PAGES

Although the health history provides important background on the child's health, the physical examination is vital to the adequate assessment of the child's condition.

Keep the following age-related considerations in mind when performing physical assessment of the pediatric patient.

Vital Signs
• Normal ranges vary with age.
• Hypotension is a late sign of shock and may not appear until circulating volume is decreased by 25% to 40%.
• Appropriate-sized cuff is essential for an accurate blood pressure reading.
• The brachial or apical site should be used for taking pulse readings in the infant or young child.
• The radial site is palpable in older children and adolescents.

Airway
• Neonates breathe through the nose.
• The airway increases in size with age.

Breathing
• Infants are diaphragmatic (abdominal) breathers.
• Ribs are pliable.
• Accessory muscles are poorly developed.

Circulation
• Stroke volume is dependent on pulse rate.
• Functional murmurs are often present.

Head and Neck
• Because the head is heavy and large, it is often injured.
• The younger the child, the heavier the head is relative to total body size.
• The musculature is weak, placing the patient at higher risk for cervical spine injuries and spinal cord trauma caused by hyperflexion or hyperextension.

Thermoregulation
- Large surface area may lose heat rapidly.
- Keep the child covered, especially an infant's head.

Growth and Development
- Infants (birth to 1 year)
  - Developing trust
  - Attached to parents
  - Minimize separation from parents
  - Older infants may localize pain
- Toddler (1 to 3 years)
  - Developing autonomy
  - Increased concerns about safety
  - Has fear of pain
- Preschoolers (3 to 6 years)
  - Learning to do things for self
  - Has ability to think magically
- School-aged child (6 to 12 years)
  - Can understand body anatomy and function
  - Wants privacy and control
- Adolescent (12 to 15 years)
  - Peer relationships are important
  - Sensitive to being different from peer group
  - Very modest

The following general considerations will facilitate the assessment.
- Illness differences in children and adults are anatomic, psychological, and physiologic.
- Treat the child and parent as one entity and try not to separate them.
- Use play therapy if time permits. Allow the child to hold a favorite toy or security object.
- Avoid sudden movement, loud noises, and other threatening behavior.
- Examine the painful areas last, when possible.
- Be honest. Tell the child if the procedure will be painful or uncomfortable.
- Protect the child's modesty and privacy.
- Explain procedures to the extent possible and according to the child's age and developmental level.

Vital Signs

The child may be allowed to sit on the parent's lap during this phase of the physical assessment. Remove or unbutton the child's shirt to observe chest movements and to listen to breath sounds.

Respiratory Rate

Count an infant's respirations by observing the movement of the abdominal wall. Respirations are mainly abdominal in an infant. Count for 1 full minute because an infant's respirations tend to be irregular. Respiratory and pulse rates decline with age. Be alert to signs of respiratory distress, including the following:

- Tachypnea
- Dysphagia and drooling, which are signs of upper airway obstruction
- Nasal flaring and accessory muscle use
- Retractions, which is a caving in of soft tissues relative to the cartilaginous and bony thorax
- Adventitious breath sounds
  - Wheezing and grunting, which are signs of lower airway obstruction
  - Barking cough and stridor, which are signs of upper airway obstruction

Be alert to the following signs and symptoms of severe hypoxia:

- Child's preference for a certain position
- Head bobbing with each breath
- Agitation or decreased level of consciousness
- Pale skin color or cyanosis (a late sign of severe hypoxia)
- Hypoventilation or apnea
- Bradycardia

PEDIATRIC RESPIRATORY RATES

AGE	RATE
Birth to 1 month	30–40
1 month to 1 year	26–40
2 to 6 years	20–30
6 to 10 years	18–24
Adolescent	16–24

Pulse Rate

The pulse is counted as you feel the wave of blood being forced through the artery. The rate varies greatly in different children of the same age and size. In a 2-year-old, the lower limit of normal is 80 and the upper limit may be 130. Normal rates also vary for teenage boys and girls. The lower limit in a 16-year-old girl is 60 and the upper limit is 100. In a boy of the same age, the limits are 55 and 95, respectively. Check the apical pulse in infants and young children; listen through the stethoscope at the apex of the heart and count the rate for 1 full minute.

Both pulse and respiratory rates are high in a neonate, but decrease gradually with age until adult values are reached.

NURSE ALERT:
Absent or weak femoral pulses may indicate coarctation of the aorta. Respiratory distress is the preceding event in most cases of pediatric cardiac arrest. Immediate attention and intervention must be given to any child with symptoms of respiratory distress.

PEDIATRIC PULSE RATES

AGE	RATE (BEATS/MINUTE)
Newborn	130
3 months	140
6 months	130
1 year	120
2 years	115
3 years	110
4 years	100
6 years	100

PEDIATRIC PULSE RATES (CONTINUED)

AGE	RATE (BEATS/MINUTE)
8 years	90
12 years	85

Blood Pressure

The pressure of the blood on the walls is a clue to the elasticity of arterial walls, peripheral vascular resistance, efficiency of the heart's pumping action, and blood volume. It is measured at the brachial, radial, popliteal, dorsalis pedis, or posterior tibial artery. Several methods are used to measure blood pressure in infants and children.

Auscultation. Using the pediatric stethoscope and cuff, measure as for an adult. The correct-sized cuff must be used. It should be long enough to encircle the extremity and should cover two thirds of the upper arm.

Subtract the diastolic reading from the systolic to determine pulse pressure, which usually varies from 20 to 50 mm Hg. Widening pulse pressure may indicate increased intracranial pressure.

Palpation. This is one of the oldest methods of measuring blood pressure. Place the cuff on the child and inflate it above the expected pressure. Put your fingers over the brachial or radial artery. Record the systolic pressure as the point where the pulse reappears; you will not be able to obtain a diastolic pressure. This is a useful method for taking the blood pressure of neonates.

Ultrasonographic (Doppler) measurement. Attach a transducer with attached cuff over an artery, usually the brachial, femoral, or popliteal artery. Inflate the cuff above the systolic pressure and gradually reduce the inflation. The transducer transmits vascular sounds, and both systolic and diastolic pressures are recorded. Measurement is by digital readout. This machine is sensitive to movement, and a child's arm must be held still to obtain an accurate reading. This device may be required to check a neonate's blood pressure.

Provide the child with an age-appropriate explanation of blood pressure measurement. Recheck the reading if there is a significant change or if an abnormal reading is obtained. Chart and report abnormal readings to the appropriate charge person.

Pressure can vary for a number of reasons. In a thigh reading, the pressure averages 10 to 20 mm Hg higher than that in an arm reading. An error in measurement can occur when the cuff is not the appropriate size. A child's blood pressure may also be affected by other factors, such as time of day, age, gender, pain, activity, medications, and emotional state.

Temperature
The child's temperature can be measured by the oral, axillary, rectal, or tympanic method. A rectal or tympanic reading may be the preferred choice for an infant or a young child, who may have difficulty holding a thermometer in the mouth or may risk injury by biting it.

The oral method of temperature measurement is the same as for adults.

For the axillary temperature, place the thermometer in the axilla and press the child's arm close to the body. The thermometer should be held in place for 5 minutes.

To take the temperature using the rectal method, place the child in a comfortable position, either on the side with knees somewhat flexed or on the stomach. Infants may be placed in the supine position with the legs held around the ankles. Insert a lubricated thermometer a maximum of 1 inch (2.5 cm) into the rectum for 3 to 5 minutes. Do not use the rectal method in a child who has had rectal surgery, is receiving chemotherapy, or may have rectal trauma.

A rectal temperature should be taken after the pulse, respiration, and blood pressure measurements because the child's reaction may influence the accuracy of those measurements.

Infrared tympanic thermometers are used in some institutions. They provide rapid results and are easier to use than conventional thermometers. Additionally, there is less exposure to infections, patients prefer them, and, unlike the oral method, the readings are not affected by eating, drinking, or smoking. The tympanic method is not recommended in infants younger than 3 months.

Slight variations in body temperature are considered normal. Be sure to document the route used. Rectal temperatures are slightly higher than oral readings, whereas axillary temperatures are slightly lower than oral readings but not the full degree Fahrenheit as once was considered. Normal temperature ranges for children are as follows:

Oral	36.4–37.4°C (97.6–99.3°F)
Rectal	37.0–37.8°C (98.6–100.0°F)
Axillary	35.8–36.6°C (96.6–98.0°F)
Tympanic	36.0–38.1°C (96.8–100.6°F)

Notify the appropriate charge person if the reading is abnormal.

NURSE ALERT:
A temperature less than 96.8°F in an infant is a significant finding that warrants attention. It may indicate sepsis or hypothermia.

Weight
Obtain an accurate record of the child's weight. It provides a means of determining progress and is essential in determining many medication dosages. Weight should be obtained in kilograms because this is the unit of measure for drug and fluid calculations.

How a child is weighed depends on the child's age. An infant is weighed naked in a warm room. Place the infant on a clean diaper or scale and record the reading while the infant is lying still. An older child is weighed in the same way as an adult. Generally, the child is weighed wearing a hospital gown. When weighing a child who is wearing a cast, be sure to note that the child has a cast and the affected limb.

Height
An infant is measured while lying on a flat surface next to a metal or wooden measuring stick. Press the infant's knees flat on the table, and measure from the top of the head to the heels with the head in the midline. Older children and adolescents may be measured while standing straight in the same manner as adults.

Head Circumference

All children under 36 months of age or those with neurologic defects should have their head circumferences measured. Place a flexible tape around the head, slightly above
the eyebrows and pinnae of the ears to the occipital promi-
nence of the skull to determine the exact measurement.

Weight, height, and head circumference should be regular-
ly plotted on approved growth charts to monitor the child's
physical development and deviations from the normal pattern. Corrections for gestational age are important when
recording measurements for children who have been born
prematurely.

Airway and Breathing

Check the airway for patency, auscultate breath sounds,
count the respiratory rate, and observe the child's color.
Observe the type of breathing, the depth and regularity of
respirations, and length of inspiration in relation to expiration.

Circulation

Observe the child's color; pallor may indicate diminished
perfusion. Auscultate for heart sounds, and evaluate the
sounds for quality, rate, intensity, and rhythm.

Measure capillary refill by applying pressure to the nail
beds or forehead, releasing and watching for circulation to
return. A delay of 3 seconds or more is abnormal.

Record the child's level of consciousness. Confusion and
lethargy may be the result of decreased perfusion to the
brain.

Assess skin turgor and check mucous membranes for
moistness. Examine the fontanelles. A sunken fontanelle
may indicate dehydration.

Evaluate peripheral pulse rate and strength. A weak
peripheral pulse may point to decreased perfusion to the
extremities.

Note the presence of bleeding and signs pointing to inter-
nal bleeding, such as a rigid abdomen.

Neurologic Status

Assess the child's level of consciousness. Is the child awake and alert, or lethargic and stuporous?

Assess the child's eye opening. Does the child look around the environment? Does the child open eyes to sound or painful stimuli only? Is there no eye opening?

Assess the child's motor response. Does the patient move spontaneously? Can he or she localize pain? Withdrawal? Is there abnormal posturing, such as decortication or decerebration? Is the child flaccid?

Assess the child's verbal response. Does the child smile, follow you with his or her eyes, recognize familiar people? Can the child be consoled, or is he or she persistently irritable, restless, or agitated? Is there no response?

Assess the size and response of pupils. Are the pupils of equal size? Do they react to light?

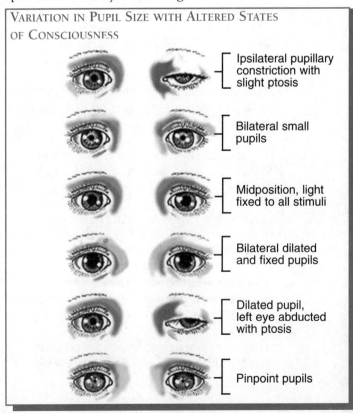

VARIATION IN PUPIL SIZE WITH ALTERED STATES OF CONSCIOUSNESS

Ipsilateral pupillary constriction with slight ptosis

Bilateral small pupils

Midposition, light fixed to all stimuli

Bilateral dilated and fixed pupils

Dilated pupil, left eye abducted with ptosis

Pinpoint pupils

A Glasgow Coma Scale adapted for pediatric use can assist in obtaining an objective assessment of neurologic status. Refer to the appendix for a pediatric Glasgow Coma Scale.

History and the child's level of consciousness are vital parts of the neurologic examination. The American Academy of Pediatrics and the American College of Emergency Physicians recommend using the AEIOU TIPS mnemonic to evaluate level of consciousness.

AEIOU TIPS TO EVALUATE ALTERED LEVEL OF CONSCIOUSNESS

CAUSE	COMMENTS
Alcohol	Found more in adolescents than in younger children
Encephalopathy	Hypertension, liver problems, Reye's syndrome
Endocrinology	Thyroid, adrenal
Electrolytes	Alterations in sodium, potassium, calcium, or magnesium levels
Insulin	Hypoglycemia, hyperglycemia
Intussusception	Decreased level of consciousness may be first indication of intussusception before abdominal symptoms appear
Overdose	Opioids and other toxins: ingested, inhaled, or transferred to fetus before birth
Uremia	Hemolytic uremic syndrome, chronic renal impairment
Trauma	One of the main causes; usually head and chest injuries leading to hypoxia
Infection	More common in children than in adults; meningitis, encephalitis, Reye's syndrome, and sepsis

AEIOU TIPS TO EVALUATE ALTERED LEVEL OF CONSCIOUSNESS
(CONTINUED)

CAUSE	COMMENTS
Psychiatric	Rare in children; consider only when other factors are ruled out
Seizure	Postictal states, syncope

Use the following AVPU mnemonic to evaluate the preverbal child:

Alert
Verbal stimuli response
Painful stimuli response
Unresponsive

Assessing Pain

Because pain is frequently the most characteristic symptom of the onset of a physical problem, it is used as a prototype for analyzing symptoms. In assessing pain, determine its type, location, severity, and duration as well as factors that cause a change in any of these: events that increase or lessen the pain, times when the pain is relieved or increased, positions that affect pain, and associated events, such as eating, stress, and coughing.

Use the following guidelines for assessing pain.
• Structure the assessment approach to the child's developmental level and personality and to the presenting circumstance.
• Obtain a pain history from the child or parents. Determine the word the child uses for pain (boo-boo, ouchee), and use it with the child in the history-taking phase of the assessment.
• Find out whether the family has any culturally determined beliefs about pain and medical care.
• Gauge the child's pain using self-report or reliable, valid, sensitive behavioral observation tools, such as smile/sad face scales, word rating scales, and 1-to-10 rating scales.
• Observe the behavior of the preverbal or nonverbal child. Use these techniques in addition to the self-report index of an older, verbal child.

Developmental Function

Assessing developmental functioning is an essential component of a complete health appraisal of the child. The Denver Developmental Screening Test (DDST) is one of the most widely used assessment instruments for children from birth through 6 years of age. However, it lacks sensitivity in identifying the child with speech and language delays and in identifying general delays in a child from a lower socioeconomic group or from a cultural background different from the norm for which the test was designed. It contains the following major classifications:

• Personal-social
• Fine motor-adaptive
• Language
• Gross motor

The Denver II is a major revision and restandardization of the original DDST. It contains a new screening manual, three additional test items, and a new interpretation of scoring.

Screening tests are effective methods of applying the knowledge of a child's expected rate of development to a large part of the population. Their success, however, is largely dependent on the expertise of the person administering them.

Explain the purpose of the test to the child and caregiver before beginning the test. It is your responsibility to ensure that caregivers know the aim and purpose of any testing or screening procedure before it is administered.

General evaluation of a child's development can be done quickly by comparing the child's age and major developmental milestones (sitting, walking, and so forth). You may find that a large, formalized screening test is impractical in most clinical settings.

Secondary Assessment

Secondary assessment begins after evaluating vital signs, airway and breathing, circulatory and neurologic systems, and developmental factors. The table below provides a head-to-toe guide to the secondary assessment of the pediatric patient.

SECONDARY ASSESSMENT OF THE PEDIATRIC PATIENT

AREA EXAMINED	WHAT TO CHECK
Head and neck	• Anterior fontanelle: open or closed • Presence of injuries and tenderness or pain • Palpate skull for hematomas or depressions • Nuchal rigidity
Eyes	• Pupils: size and reaction to light • Tearing • Deviation • Draining and periorbital swelling • Sclera: presence of jaundice

Ears	• Drainage
	  - Clear drainage: cerebrospinal fluid with a basilar skull fracture
	  - Purulent or bloody drainage: otitis media

Nose	• Ecchymosis (Battle's sign): basilar skull fracture • Nasal flaring: increased respiratory effort • Drainage (clear): cerebrospinal fluid in presence of basilar skull fracture • Foul odor: presence of a foreign body
Throat **!** **NURSE ALERT:** Defer this part of the examination if the child is experiencing severe respiratory distress.	• Swelling or exudates in pharynx • Cervical lymph glands: swelling
Mouth	• Color of oral mucosa • Presence of lesions • Moistness of lips and mucous membranes

SECONDARY ASSESSMENT OF THE PEDIATRIC PATIENT
(CONTINUED)

AREA EXAMINED	WHAT TO CHECK
Chest	• Respiratory status as found during primary assessment • Presence of rashes or bruising • Presence of tenderness
Abdomen	• Distention; if severe, may compromise the airway because of pressure on the diaphragm • Abdominal girth • Bowel sounds • Tenderness • Ecchymosis
Genitalia and rectum **!** **NURSE ALERT:** This assessmemt may be conducted when rectal temperature is taken or it may be deferred.	• Diaper rash • Vaginal discharge or irritation • Odor • Rectal bleeding or tears • Discharge from penis • Trauma
Extremities and skin	Compare bilaterally for: • Swelling • Movement (range of motion) • Deformities • Sensation • Strength • Pulses • Bruises or rashes • Color

Other aspects in the secondary assessment to consider are the following:
• Don't focus on the obvious.
• Consider any chronic condition when assessing.

- Always listen to the parents or caregivers and ask for their opinions of the child's condition.
- Be alert to signs of child abuse and know what your responsibility is in reporting abuse.

Documentation must be accurate and complete. Although documentation will focus on any chief complaint or problem, all collateral findings and interventions must be documented as well. Be sure to record the following:
- Time of examination
- Presenting problem or chief complaint
- General appearance of the child
- Initial assessment, including vital signs
- Interventions and the child's response
- Planned follow-up and instructions given
- Condition on discharge

Note that some of the elements above are pertinent to emergency department situations.

The complexity of a child's mental and physical health can never be completely measured by any one index. To evaluate the child's total well-being requires evaluating data from a comprehensive history, physical examination, and developmental screening.

Suggested Readings

Bates, B. *A Guide to Physical Examination and History Taking.* 5th ed. Philadelphia: J. B. Lippincott, 1991.

Chamberlain, J. M., and T. E. Ferndrup. "The Ears Have It: Using and Interpreting Tympanic Thermometers." *Advance for Nurse Practitioners* 3 (February 1995): 29–32.

Curry, D. M., and J. C. Duby. "Developmental Surveillance by Pediatric Nurses." *Pediatric Nursing* 20 (January/February 1994): 40–44.

Gerchufsky, M. "A Closer Look at Contraindication Myths: To Immunize or Not to Immunize." *Advance for Nurse Practitioners* 3 (February 1995): 33–34, 47.

Stroud, T. "Airway, Breathing, Circulation and Disability: What Is Different About Kids?" *Journal of Emergency Nursing* 18 (April 1992): 107–116.

SECTION III. SYSTEMIC REVIEW

Chapter 5. Head and Neck
▽ ▽ ▽ ▽ ▽ ▽ ▽

Introduction

SEE TEXT PAGES

Many of the common problems that cause parents or care-givers to bring children for medical attention are found in the head and neck. They include the common cold, pharyngitis, otitis externa, and otitis media. Consequently, health care providers who treat children spend the most time managing ear, nose, and throat problems.

Overview: Common Infections

Most common infections of the head and neck are caused by viral infections of the upper respiratory tract: respiratory syncytial virus, rhinovirus influenza, parainfluenza, and adenoviruses.

Tonsillitis is an inflammation of the tonsils and their crypts that is usually caused by a virus or streptococcal organism. Tonsillectomy may be considered for a child who has frequent episodes of tonsillitis or who has had a peritonsillar abscess.

Adenoiditis is an inflammation of the adenoids, which are lymphoid tissue structures located on the posterior wall of the nasopharynx. Adenoidectomy is a consideration for the child who has recurrent otitis media, severe nasal obstruction, dentofacial deformity associated with adenoid hypertrophy, or persistent upper airway infections with mouth breathing and snoring.

Tonsillectomy and adenoidectomy are the most common major surgical procedures performed on children in the United States. Controversy exists about the necessity of these procedures. They are frequently done as one procedure, and many are performed on an out-patient basis. Patients may experience significant postoperative pain, and there is a risk that potentially serious complications, such as airway obstruction and hemorrhage, may develop.

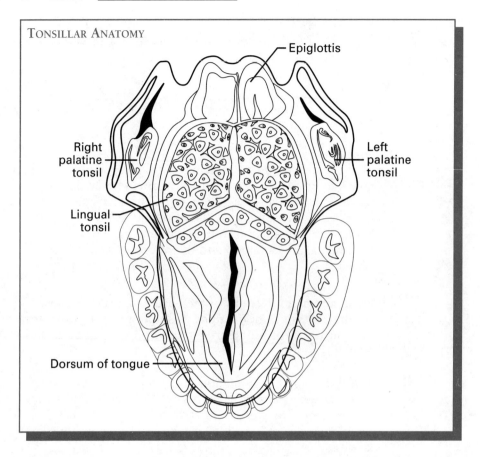

TONSILLAR ANATOMY

Epiglottis

Right palatine tonsil

Left palatine tonsil

Lingual tonsil

Dorsum of tongue

NURSING DIAGNOSIS: INEFFECTIVE AIRWAY CLEARANCE

RELATED TO:
• *Nasal secretions secondary to the common cold*

Nursing Interventions	Rationales
• Encourage the use of a humidifier.	• To increase ambient humidity to help liquefy thick nasal secretions
• Perform nasal aspiration, if required.	• To clear nasal secretions

COLLABORATIVE MANAGEMENT

Interventions	Rationales
• Administer medications as ordered: decongestant nasal drops or oral medications.	• To encourage drying of nasal secretions

NURSE ALERT:
Saline nasal drops are recommended to liquefy nasal secretions in the young child or infant. Decongestants must be used with care in this age-group.

OUTCOME:	EVALUATION CRITERIA:
• The child will experience decreased nasal secretions.	• The child is able to maintain a clear upper airway. • The child is able to maintain adequate oral intake.

NURSING DIAGNOSIS: HIGH RISK FOR INFECTION

RELATED TO:
• *Pharyngitis, tonsillitis, adenoiditis*

Nursing Interventions	Rationales
• Obtain throat culture results.	• To identify pathogen causing infection

COLLABORATIVE MANAGEMENT

Interventions	Rationales
• Administer antibiotic therapy, as prescribed.	• To reduce infection

OUTCOME:	EVALUATION CRITERIA:
• The child will be free of signs of infection.	• Tissue edema is absent or decreased. • Vital signs are normal. • Laboratory values are normal.

NURSING DIAGNOSIS: PAIN

RELATED TO:

• *Inflammation of tonsillar, adenoidal, or pharyngeal tissue*

Nursing Interventions	Rationales
• Apply ice packs to the child's throat.	• To promote comfort
• Recommend that the older child use throat lozenges or spray.	• To promote comfort

COLLABORATIVE MANAGEMENT

Interventions	Rationales
• Administer medications, as ordered: analgesics, antipyretics.	• To reduce infection and fever causing discomfort

OUTCOME:

• The child will experience reduced discomfort.

EVALUATION CRITERIA:

• The child reports an increase in comfort.

• The child's temperature remains normal.

NURSING DIAGNOSIS: INEFFECTIVE AIRWAY CLEARANCE

RELATED TO:

• *Postoperative bleeding, difficulty swallowing and clearing secretions*

Nursing Interventions	Rationales
• Place the child partly on his or her side and abdomen, flexing the knee of the top leg to hold the position.	• To facilitate drainage of secretions
• Observe the child for signs of increasing distress, such as regurgitation and gurgling.	• To anticipate the child's need for assistance in clearing secretions
• Encourage the child to expectorate blood or mucus gently.	• To facilitate drainage of secretions

COLLABORATIVE MANAGEMENT

Interventions
- Cauterize or ligate bleeding tissues.

Rationales
- To control bleeding

OUTCOME:
- The child will maintain a patent airway and will adequately manage secretions.

EVALUATION CRITERIA:
- The child maintains normal respiratory effort.
- The child can clear his or her own secretions.

NURSING DIAGNOSIS: DECREASED CARDIAC OUTPUT

RELATED TO:
- *Postoperative hemorrhage*

Nursing Interventions
- Monitor the child for signs of bleeding.

- Watch for signs of hemorrhage, such as:
  - excessive swallowing
  - pallor
  - tachycardia
  - increased capillary refill time
  - lethargy.

Rationales
- To identify early signs of decreased cardiac output and provide appropriate interventions

- To identify potentially life-threatening conditions and provide appropriate interventions

COLLABORATIVE MANAGEMENT

Interventions
- Apply packing, as ordered.
- Assist with ligation procedures.
- Administer I.V. fluids, as ordered.

Rationales
- To prevent hemorrhage
- To prevent hemorrhage
- To replace loss of volume and ensure adequate hydration

NURSING DIAGNOSIS: DECREASED CARDIAC OUTPUT
(CONTINUED)

OUTCOME:
- The child will maintain adequate cardiac output and bleeding from the surgical site will be under control.

EVALUATION CRITERIA:
- Capillary refill time is within normal limits.

- Vital signs are normal.

- The child has normal skin color and turgor.

- Bleeding is reduced or stopped.

NURSING DIAGNOSIS: PAIN

RELATED TO:
- *Operative procedure*

Nursing Interventions
- Apply an ice pack to the child's throat.

- Encourage the caregivers to comfort the child.

Rationales
- To reduce swelling and discomfort

- To relieve the child's distress

COLLABORATIVE MANAGEMENT

Interventions
- Administer medications, as ordered: acetaminophen.

Rationales
- To alleviate discomfort

OUTCOME:
- The child will experience reduced or absent pain.

EVALUATION CRITERIA:
- The child reports decreased or absent pain.

- Vital signs are normal.

- There are no obvious signs of pain or discomfort, such as facial grimacing or crying.

Patient Teaching

Before the surgery, explain the procedure clearly and completely to the caregiver and to the child, if appropriate.

Instruct the caregiver not to give aspirin to the child and to report any of the following signs to the health care provider:
• Bright red bleeding
• Frequent swallowing, which may indicate that the child is swallowing blood
• Temperature higher than 100°F (37.8°C)
• Pain unrelieved by acetaminophen with codeine

Instruct the caregiver to keep the child quiet for a few days. Advise the caregiver to give the child small, frequent sips of fluid and then proceed to a soft diet after fluids are well tolerated. Emphasize the need to provide nourishing fluids and soft foods.

Recommend that the child continue with a regular nap or rest period during convalescence.

Stress the need to protect the child from exposure to infections.

Documentation

• Vital signs, especially during the postoperative period
• Blood loss, including frequency of swallowing
• Signs of decreased cardiac output:
  - Level of consciousness
  - Capillary refill time
  - Peripheral pulse quality

Overview: Epistaxis

Epistaxis, or nosebleed, is a frightening experience for many children, although most nosebleeds are benign and do not pose an immediate threat. Bleeding from the nose can occur either anteriorly or posteriorly. Significant epistaxis in children usually occurs in association with increased pressure from secretions in the nose caused by respiratory tract infection, allergies, sinusitis, nose picking or blowing, local trauma, a foreign body, overly dry air, septal deviation, or nasal fractures. Anterior epistaxis is most common; posterior epistaxis is usually seen only in the elderly patient.

NURSING DIAGNOSIS: HIGH RISK FOR FLUID VOLUME DEFICIT

RELATED TO:
• *Nasal hemorrhage*

Nursing Interventions	Rationales
• Assess vital signs. Be alert to signs of shock.	• To identify signs of impending severe hemorrhage
• Position the child in an upright position with the head bent slightly forward.	• To lower venous pressure and facilitate expectoration of blood
• Apply firm pressure by compressing the anterior aspect of the nose between the thumb and forefinger at least 5 minutes. Sometimes it is recommended that all clots be evacuated before applying pressure.	• To reduce perfusion through the anterior ethmoid artery
• Place ice packs on the bridge of the child's nose. Use gauze or a washcloth to prevent dripping.	• To promote local vasoconstriction and cessation of bleeding
• Suction the child's nose if bleeding continues after 10 minutes of pressure.	• To remove blood causing nasal obstruction

COLLABORATIVE MANAGEMENT

Interventions	Rationales
• Apply a topical anesthetic and vasoconstrictor, as ordered.	• To shrink nasal mucosa and decrease blood flow
• Apply silver nitrate stick directly to bleeding point, as ordered.	• To cauterize source of bleeding
• Place a cotton ball impregnated with cocaine or a half-and-half mixture of 2% tetracaine and 1% phenylephrine into bleeding nostril spectrum using a nasal speculum or bayonet forceps, as ordered.	• To reduce pain, promote local vasoconstriction by shrinking nasal mucosa, and decrease bleeding

COLLABORATIVE MANAGEMENT (CONTINUED)

Interventions (Continued)	Rationales (Continued)
• Apply anterior nasal packing for bleeding that is not controlled by coagulation. Note that this requires antibiotic prophylaxis with ampicillin, tetracycline, or a cephalosporin.	• To control bleeding and reduce adverse effects on mucociliary clearance caused by the packing that may lead to bacterial superinfection
• If necessary, assist with surgical vessel ligation of the anterior ethmoid artery or external carotid artery.	• To stop uncontrolled hemorrhage

NURSE ALERT:
Severe blood loss, which may cause shock, should be treated with I.V. fluids or blood administration to compensate for volume loss that often accompanies hemorrhagic shock.

OUTCOME:	EVALUATION CRITERIA:
• The child will maintain adequate circulating blood volume.	• Bleeding from the nose is decreased or stopped.
	• Vital signs are normal.
	• The child shows no signs of shock.
	• The child's color, appearance, and behavior return to normal.

NURSING DIAGNOSIS: ANXIETY

RELATED TO:
• *Fears about the child's blood loss*

Nursing Interventions	Rationales
• Assess the caregivers' and child's anxiety related to the hemorrhage and fear of treatment and outcome.	• To focus your interventions on the specific causes of anxiety and reassure the patient and the caregiver that feelings of anxiety are normal
• Provide discharge instructions and information about follow-up examinations, if necessary.	• To reduce anxiety
• Provide reassurance in a calm manner with a positive attitude.	• To reduce anxiety

COLLABORATIVE MANAGEMENT

Interventions	Rationales
• Provide information regarding medical interventions, such as nasal packing and cauterization, and surgical interventions.	• To inform the caregiver and the child about treatment plans

OUTCOME:	EVALUATION CRITERIA:
• The patient and his or her caregivers will demonstrate a decrease in anxiety level.	• The child and the caregivers remain calm and cooperative.
	• The caregiver comforts the child as appropriate.

Patient Teaching

Instruct the caregivers about care of nasal packing when the child is sent home with a nasal pack. Emphasize that the child should keep his or her head elevated and avoid straining and blowing out the pack.

Explain antibiotic and analgesic administration.

Instruct the patient and caregivers how to control future epistaxis.

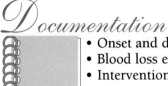

Documentation

- Onset and duration of epistaxis
- Blood loss estimate
- Interventions and patient response

Overview: Acute Otitis Externa

Most cases of otitis externa, "swimmer's ear," are not serious, although the condition can be painful.

NURSING DIAGNOSIS: PAIN

RELATED TO:
- *Infection of the ear tissues*

Nursing Interventions	Rationales
• Assess pain using age-appropriate tools for objective measurements.	• To quantify response to interventions for pain
• Apply warm compresses to the child's ear.	• To provide comfort
• Assist the child to assume a comfortable position.	• To increase comfort
• Speak slowly and clearly while facing the patient.	• To ensure that the child can hear your instructions
• Instruct the patient and his or her caregivers about the need to avoid swimming until the infection has been resolved.	• To provide sufficient time for healing

NURSING DIAGNOSIS: PAIN (CONTINUED)

COLLABORATIVE MANAGEMENT

Interventions
- Administer medications, as ordered: analgesics, antibiotics, antipyretics.

Rationales
- To reduce infection and pain and control fever

NURSE ALERT:
When administering ear drops, instruct the child to lie on one side while the drops are instilled and to remain in that position for at least 5 minutes.

OUTCOME:
- The child will experience reduced pain or discomfort.

EVALUATION CRITERIA:
- The child reports the absence or reduction of pain.

- The child displays no outward signs of pain, such as facial grimacing or crying.

Patient Teaching

Instruct the caregivers about the importance of completing the entire course of antibiotic therapy to fully resolve the infection. Explain the need to avoid swimming until the infection has been resolved. Suggest that a child who gets "swimmer's ear" repeatedly may benefit from routine rinsing of the ear canals at bedtime.

Documentation

- Child's response to treatment
- Medications administered

Overview: Acute Otitis Media

One of the most prevalent diseases of childhood, otitis media effects about 70% of all children by the age of 3. The infection is more common in children who reside in households with many members or with smokers. There is also a familial tendency for acute otitis media.

NURSING DIAGNOSIS: PAIN

RELATED TO:
- *Infection and fever associated with acute otitis media*

Nursing Interventions	Rationales
• Assess pain using age-appropriate tools for objective measurements.	• To quantify response to interventions for pain
• Apply warm compresses to the child's ear.	• To provide comfort
• Assist the child to assume a comfortable position.	• To increase comfort
• Speak slowly and clearly while facing the patient.	• To ensure that the child can hear your instructions

COLLABORATIVE MANAGEMENT

Interventions	Rationales
• Administer medications, as ordered: analgesics, antibiotics, antipyretics.	• To reduce infection and pain and control fever

NURSE ALERT:
When administering ear drops, instruct the child to lie on one side while the drops are instilled and to remain in that position for at least 5 minutes.

• Instruct the caregivers to bring the child in for a follow-up examination within 2 weeks of initial intervention. Complete resolution of the condition should occur in 6 weeks.	• To ensure adequate follow-up care

NURSING DIAGNOSIS: PAIN *(CONTINUED)*

COLLABORATIVE MANAGEMENT *(CONTINUED)*

Interventions *(Continued)*

- Consult with the health care provider about the need for surgical tympanotomy tubes. Explain the procedure to the caregivers and the child.

Rationales *(Continued)*

- To provide additional options for ensuring drainage and ventilation of the middle ear

OUTCOME:

- The child will experience reduced pain or discomfort.

EVALUATION CRITERIA:

- The child reports the absence or reduction of pain.

- The child displays no outward signs of pain, such as facial grimacing or crying.

Patient Teaching

Instruct the caregivers about the importance of maintaining the child in an upright position after feedings.

Encourage the child to blow his or her nose gently. Teach the older child the Valsalva maneuver. Children who can safely chew gum or blow up balloons can usually perform this maneuver adequately.

Documentation

- Child's response to treatment
- Medications administered

Chapter 6. Respiratory System

▽　▽　▽　▽　▽　▽　▽

Introduction

SEE TEXT PAGES

A child's upper airway differs from an adult's airway in a number of ways.
• The larynx is somewhat anterior.
• The epiglottis is U-shaped and extends into the pharynx.
• The vocal cords are short and concave.
• In children younger than 8 years of age, the narrowest section of the airway is at the cricoid cartilage located below the vocal cords.

Any respiratory disease may cause obstruction of a child's airway because of the airway's size and position. Minimal edema in the slender area below the cricoid cartilage may produce respiratory distress and stridor.

In the infant and young child, the lower airway is small and the supporting cartilage is not as developed as that in the adult, making it more easily obstructed by mucus, blood, pus, edema, foreign bodies, or constriction.

Other factors leading to respiratory distress in children include the following:
• The ribs are more compliant.
• The mediastinum is thinner and more mobile.
• Infants are nose-breathers.
• Children rely on the diaphragm for adequate chest expansion.
• Metabolic rate and oxygen consumption are much higher than in adults.
• Airway resistance in infants is 15 times greater than in adults.
• A child's accessory muscles of inspiration tire quickly because of less reserve muscle glycogen.

Respiratory disorders are the most common cause of illness in infants and children. Although most respiratory disorders are mild and resolve without medical treatment, some acute infections rapidly advance to respiratory obstruction and failure. Diseases that affect the respiratory system pose the greatest threat to children. The following are examples

of respiratory diseases and infections that affect children:
• Bronchiolitis
• Laryngotracheobronchitis (croup)
• Epiglottiditis
• Acute asthma

Planning and interventions for general respiratory emergencies begin with determining priorities: control and maintenance of airway, breathing, and circulation. Next, a nursing care plan must be developed that is tailored to the specific condition. Finally, any necessary equipment and supplies must be obtained and readied.

Overview: Epiglottiditis

Epiglottiditis occurs most often during the winter and spring months; its peak incidence is in children aged 2 to 7 years. Acute epiglottiditis, a life-threatening condition, is characterized by edema of the epiglottis and aryepiglottic folds not extending beneath the vocal cords. The child often assumes a "tripod" or "sniffing" position, with mouth-breathing, drooling, and a foreboding, tired facial appearance. This is a true medical emergency that requires personnel skilled in pediatric airway management. Airway access can be best obtained in an operating room with the child under anesthesia and in the presence of an ear, nose, and throat (ENT) surgeon if a surgical airway should be required.

Vaccinating children less than 1 year old with *Haemophilus* vaccine reduces the incidence of acute epiglottiditis.

NURSING DIAGNOSES: IMPAIRED GAS EXCHANGE
INEFFECTIVE AIRWAY CLEARANCE

RELATED TO:
• *Laryngospasm, edema, and restricted air flow*

Nursing Interventions	Rationales
• Encourage the caregiver to remain with the child and to comfort him or her, as needed.	• To avoid increasing the child's anxiety, which could lead to life-threatening laryngospasms, and to decrease crying, which can increase oxygen demands

Nursing Interventions (Continued)

- Position the child to facilitate breathing, and provide humidified "blow-by" oxygen.

- Obtain arterial blood gas levels and pulse oximetry values.

- Monitor for cardiac arrhythmia secondary to alterations in arterial blood gas levels.

- Prepare the child for emergency endotracheal (ET) intubation, cricothyroidotomy, or tracheostomy. The child may need a smaller ET tube than normal as a result of edema.

- Prepare for aggressive ventilatory support with bag-valve-mask followed by ventilator when the airway is secured.

- Delay diagnostic procedures, except lateral neck radiograph, until epiglottiditis is ruled out or airway is secured.

Rationales (Continued)

- To ease breathing efforts and provide additional oxygen in a noninvasive manner

- To identify the potential for impaired gas exchange

- To detect hypoxia as indicated by bradyarrhythmias

- To provide an airway

- To ensure adequate ventilation

- To avoid agitation, which can cause laryngospasms

COLLABORATIVE MANAGEMENT

Interventions

- Consult with personnel trained in pediatric airway management, including anesthesia and ENT.

Rationales

- To determine if intubation is required and to ensure that the procedure is correctly carried out

NURSE ALERT:
The surgical team does not insert I.V. lines or stimulate the throat in any way until the child is sufficiently anesthetized to avoid triggering laryngospasm.

NURSING DIAGNOSIS: IMPAIRED GAS EXCHANGE *(CONTINUED)*

COLLABORATIVE MANAGEMENT *(CONTINUED)*

Interventions *(Continued)*

- Establish I.V. access after airway has been secured.

- Administer medications, as ordered: I.V. ampicillin, chloramphenicol, cephalosporin antibiotic, dexamethasone, sedatives.

- Assist with extubation procedures. Monitor the child's condition closely for signs of edema.

Rationales *(Continued)*

- To provide route for administration of medications

- To reduce airway edema, resolve underlying infection, and ensure that the child remains still to avoid accidental extubation

- To ensure a patent airway

NURSE ALERT:
Extubation is normally done once airway edema has diminished. Be alert to signs of increasing edema that will make reintubation more difficult.

- Explain the required 10-day, postextubation antibiotic regimen.

- To ensure patient and caregiver compliance and promote complete resolution of the infection

OUTCOME:

- The child will maintain adequate ventilation and gas exchange and be free of infection.

EVALUATION CRITERIA:

- Respiratory rate and effort are normal.

- The child's skin is of normal color and there is no sign of cyanosis.

- Edema of the upper airways is decreased or absent.

- Arterial blood gas values and pulse oximetry indicate normal gas exchange.

Patient Teaching

Explain all ongoing procedures to the patient and the parents or other caregivers.

Encourage the caregiver to play an active role in supporting the child throughout all procedures, particularly during the acute phase, to reduce the child's anxiety.

Documentation

• Ongoing respiratory assessment
• Interventions and response to interventions

Overview: Croup

Infectious laryngotracheobronchitis, the proper name for croup, is common in the fall and winter months. It generally affects children between the ages of 6 months and 2 years and is more prevalent in boys than in girls. An inflammation of the larynx and subglottic area, croup is not usually a life-threatening condition and is most often managed at home; in some cases, it may require hospitalization.

NURSING DIAGNOSIS: INEFFECTIVE AIRWAY CLEARANCE

RELATED TO:
• *Edema and potential obstruction of the upper airway*

Nursing Interventions	Rationales
• Monitor vital signs closely, including the pattern, rate, and characteristics of respirations. Be alert for signs of increasing airway obstruction, such as: - tachycardia - tachypnea - positions for mouth-breathing - retractions or stridor at rest - pallor - listlessness - circumoral cyanosis - anxiety - restlessness - diminished breath sounds.	• To identify trends that indicate increasing respiratory distress

NURSING DIAGNOSIS: INEFFECTIVE AIRWAY CLEARANCE
(CONTINUED)

Nursing Interventions (Continued)

- Note and record clinical features of the child's condition:
  - color
  - wheezing
  - nasal flaring
  - hoarseness
  - drooling
  - cough qualities
  - location and type of pain.

- Prepare emergency equipment.

- Provide humidified oxygen or room air cool mist.

- Monitor pulse oximetry and the effects of humidified oxygen at the flow rate ordered.

- Assist the child to maintain an upright position or a position of comfort.

- Ensure a quiet, calm environment and take measures to minimize the child's crying.

Rationales (Continued)

- To document the patient's condition for tracking the effectiveness of interventions

- To assist with ventilation and intubation, if required

- To decrease edema and provide supplemental oxygen

- To ensure adequate oxygenation

- To increase respiratory excursion

- To reduce stress and related oxygen demands

COLLABORATIVE MANAGEMENT

Interventions

- Treat the severely distressed child with racemic epinephrine by nebulizer, as ordered.

- Administer antibiotics, as ordered, to the child with prolonged episodes of croup or to the child transferred from another health care facility.

Rationales

- To decrease upper airway edema

- To reduce the risk of infection

COLLABORATIVE MANAGEMENT *(CONTINUED)*

Interventions *(Continued)*

- Administer sedation, if ordered, to the child who is intubated.

NURSE ALERT:
A child who requires racemic epi-nephrine treatment should be admitted to the hospital for obser-vation.

- Administer steroids, as ordered.

OUTCOME:

- The child will appear comfort-able and maintain adequate ven-tilation and oxygenation.

Rationales *(Continued)*

- To reduce the risk of extubation

- To reduce airway edema

EVALUATION CRITERIA:

- Respiratory rate and effort are nor-mal.

- There is no cyanosis.

- The use of accessory muscles to aid respiration has been dimin-ished or stopped.

NURSING DIAGNOSIS: ANXIETY

RELATED TO:
- *Dyspnea, unfamiliar environment, interventions, and care equipment*

Nursing Interventions

- Orient the child to time, place, and physical status, as appropriate.

- Allow the parents or caregivers to remain with the child.

- Explain the purpose of the equipment to be used, such as X-ray and oxygen equipment, using appropriate language for the child's age and developmen-tal level.

Rationales

- To familiarize the child with the environment

- To prevent distress and crying, which can lead to laryngospasm and further airway obstruction

- To reduce anxiety and increase patient knowledge

NURSING DIAGNOSIS: ANXIETY (CONTINUED)

COLLABORATIVE MANAGEMENT

Interventions

• Emphasize the need for all members of the health care team to approach the child slowly, in a nonthreatening manner.

Rationales

• To avoid startling the child and increasing his or her anxiety

OUTCOME:

• The child will demonstrate reduced anxiety.

EVALUATION CRITERIA:

• The child's rest and sleep patterns are normal.

• The child expresses, in a developmentally appropriate manner, a reduction in feelings of anxiety.

• The caregivers provide comfort to the child.

Patient Teaching

Provide instruction about the home management of mild croup.
• Use a cool humidifier or take the child into the bathroom and run the shower when the child has breathing difficulties.
• Provide additional oral fluids.
• Provide the child with quiet activities with frequent rest periods as needed.

Provide information that will help the caregivers identify signs of increasing respiratory distress.

Instruct the caregivers in the use of medications, as prescribed, such as oral steroids and antipyretics.

Documentation

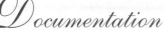

• Patient respiratory status, especially stridor, retractions, and breath sounds
• Patient response to therapy
• Vital signs, especially respiratory rate, pattern, and effort

Overview: Asthma

An obstructive pulmonary disease, asthma is the most common chronic illness in children, with 10% to 20% of children being affected at some time. It is more common in males until puberty; then it is more common in females.

NURSING DIAGNOSES: IMPAIRED GAS EXCHANGE
INEFFECTIVE AIRWAY CLEARANCE

RELATED TO:
- *Bronchospasm, edema, and elevated airway mucus production*

Nursing Interventions	Rationales
• Position the patient in high Fowler's position.	• To facilitate breathing
• Assist the patient in removal of secretions by deep breathing and coughing.	• To mobilize secretions
• Administer fluids by the I.V. route if the child is unable to tolerate fluid intake by the oral route.	• To liquefy secretions
• Establish and maintain I.V. access in severe exacerbations of illness.	• To provide access for medications and fluids
• Communicate frequently with the child and caregivers to explain all procedures in a calm and reassuring manner. Encourage the caregiver to remain with the child.	• To reduce anxiety and alleviate stress
• For the child experiencing a severe attack, monitor ECG for cardiac arrhythmias secondary to hypoxia or acidosis.	• To identify conditions that may require emergency intervention
• Monitor the child's response to medication.	• To evaluate the effectiveness of the medication
• Continually monitor pulse oximetry.	• To ensure adequate oxygenation

NURSING DIAGNOSES: IMPAIRED GAS EXCHANGE (CONTINUED)

Nursing Interventions *(Continued)*

- Monitor arterial blood gas levels.

- Prepare for more aggressive ventilatory support, if required.

Rationales *(Continued)*

- To ensure adequate ventilation and oxygenation

- To ensure adequate respiration

COLLABORATIVE MANAGEMENT

Interventions

- Administer supplemental oxygen, based on pulse oximetry and arterial blood gas levels.

- Administer medications, as ordered: aerosolized bronchodilators, steroids.

- Administer I.V. or oral corticosteroids, as ordered.

Rationales

- To maintain tissue perfusion

- To treat bronchospasms and reduce edema

- To decrease airway edema

OUTCOME:

- The child will maintain adequate tissue perfusion and experience decreased bronchospasm.

EVALUATION CRITERIA:

- Breath sounds are bilateral and even.

- Adventitious breath sounds are diminished or absent.

- The child can mobilize and expectorate secretions.

- Respiratory rate and depth are normal.

- The use of accessory muscles to aid respiration has been diminished or stopped.

- The child rests comfortably in a relaxed body position with no signs of distress, such as facial grimacing.

NURSING DIAGNOSES: IMPAIRED GAS EXCHANGE (CONTINUED)

OUTCOME: *(CONTINUED)*

- The child will maintain adequate tissue perfusion and experience decreased bronchospasm. *(continued)*

EVALUATION CRITERIA: *(CONTINUED)*

- Arterial blood gas levels are normal.

- The child's skin and mucous membrane color is normal.

Patient Teaching

Educate the child, family, and other caregivers regarding discharge instructions and follow-up treatment and evaluations.

Explain the disease process, aggravating allergens, precipitating factors, and medications (reason, route, dose, and side effects).

Emphasize that corticosteroid therapy must never be discontinued abruptly; it must be tapered off as prescribed.

Explain the importance of hydration, avoidance of allergens, use of home nebulizers and peak flowmeters, relaxation techniques, and controlled breathing.

Identify the signs and symptoms of increased distress and when to seek medical intervention.

Documentation

- Medication prescribed and patient response
- Patient response to interventions
- Vital signs, especially respiratory rate, pattern, and effort as well as breath sounds and skin color

Overview: Respiratory Syncytial Virus

Respiratory syncytial virus (RSV) is a ubiquitous human pathogen that produces a wide variety of respiratory diseases in all age-groups and is responsible for most cases of bronchiolitis and viral pneumonia. It is the most significant respiratory pathogen in infants and young children and a major cause of serious lower respiratory tract infection in children under 1 year of age.

Respiratory syncytial virus is the causative organism in 5% to 40% of pneumonia cases and 50% to 90% of bronchiolitis cases, which occur most often in the first year of life. The virus persists later in life as a pathogen responsible for tracheobronchitis and exacerbations of reactive airway disease.

Respiratory syncytial virus is present in all geographic and climatic areas but has a distinctive seasonal profile in the United States, where it produces an outbreak each winter that extends into spring.

NURSING DIAGNOSES: IMPAIRED GAS EXCHANGE
INEFFECTIVE AIRWAY CLEARANCE

RELATED TO:
- *Infection by the respiratory syncytial virus*

Nursing Interventions	Rationales
• Provide adequate hydration.	• To promote liquefication of thick secretions
• Monitor infants younger than 3 months of age for signs of apnea.	• To identify signs of apnea and provide early intervention
• Suction the child's nasopharynx, as necessary.	• To clear upper airway
• Monitor the child's condition carefully.	• To identify signs of respiratory compromise and dehydration

COLLABORATIVE MANAGEMENT

Interventions	Rationales
• Provide oxygen therapy, as needed, for hypoxia.	• To ensure adequate oxygenation
• Administer aerosolized ribavirin, as ordered.	• To improve the clinical course of bronchiolitis and pneumonia in high-risk populations

COLLABORATIVE MANAGEMENT (CONTINUED)

Interventions (Continued)
- Administer aerosolized bronchodilators, as needed.

Rationales (Continued)
- To provide relief from respiratory distress

NURSE ALERT:
Although the use of bronchodilators is controversial, some recommend a trial in infants over 6 months of age.

OUTCOME:
- The child will maintain adequate ventilation and respiration.

EVALUATION CRITERIA:
- The upper airway is free of secretions.
- Respiratory effort is normal.
- Oxygen saturation is within normal limits.

Patient Teaching

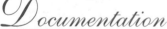

Explain procedures and interventions to parents or caregivers.

Children who are well enough to be discharged may have residual symptoms for several days. Teach parents or caregivers how to recognize increased distress.

Documentation

- Thorough respiratory assessment
- Response to bronchodilators, if used
- Rapid RSV screening results

Nursing Research

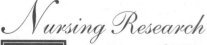

Because rapid RSV screening is currently available, future nursing research may be revised regarding the impact early screening measures have on nosocomial spread of RSV infection. Such screening enables the RSV status to be identified early in hospitalization.

Chapter 7. Cardiovascular System

▽   ▽   ▽   ▽   ▽   ▽   ▽

Introduction

SEE TEXT PAGES

Most children are born with strong hearts. As fetal circulation converts to postnatal circulation, the system begins to operate in the same manner as the adult cardiovascular system, with parameters for normal rates and pressures changing with growth.

Overview: Arrhythmias

The cardiac conduction system paces the heart, generating impulses to stimulate contraction. An arrhythmia exists when there is interference with any part of the cycle. Rhythm disturbances are seldom primary events in children but usually result from some disease state or clinical condition.

Arrhythmias may occur during or after cardiovascular surgery, either as a result of direct trauma to the conduction tissue or because of edema and other inflammatory responses near the structures.

Bradyarrhythmia

A persistent heart rate of less than 100 beats per minute in an infant and less than 80 beats per minute in a child is considered bradycardia. Always evaluate the child's heart rate in light of his or her appearance, condition, and activity level. A rate of 50 beats per minute may be normal in an athletic adolescent, whereas a heart rate of 100 beats per minute is probably too slow in a seriously ill child or toddler.

In general, bradyarrhythmias, which adversely affect cardiac output, should be managed initially by establishing and ensuring adequate ventilation and oxygenation. Pharmacologic interventions, such as the administration of atropine and sympathomimetics, may also be used. The use of cardiac pacing may be considered.

NURSING DIAGNOSIS: DECREASED CARDIAC OUTPUT

RELATED TO:
• *Bradyarrhythmia*

Nursing Interventions	Rationales

• Assess the child's:
  - skin color and temperature
  - capillary refill time
  - peripheral pulses
  - level of consciousness.
	• To determine the effectiveness of cardiac output

• Apply a cardiac monitor.	• To provide ongoing data about cardiac rhythm by way of continuous ECG tracings
• Assess the adequacy of the child's ventilation. Provide supplemental high-flow oxygen if the child has adequate respiratory effort.	• To treat hypoxia, which is a common cause of bradycardia
• Assist with ventilation by way of a bag-valve-mask device and high-flow oxygen.	• To treat hypoxia, which is a common cause of bradycardia
• Perform bag-valve-mask ventilation and external chest compressions if the child is without spontaneous respiration and there is evidence of insufficient cardiac output.	• To treat significant bradycardia as a terminal rhythm
• Establish I.V. access.	• To infuse drugs and fluids as necessary
• If the child is experiencing hypothermia, warm the child using warming lights.	• To correct hypothermia

COLLABORATIVE MANAGEMENT

Interventions	Rationales
• Administer medications, as ordered: atropine, epinephrine.	• To accelerate inherent pacemaker and conduction and to increase heart rate and contractility

NURSING DIAGNOSIS: DECREASED CARDIAC OUTPUT
(CONTINUED)

COLLABORATIVE MANAGEMENT *(CONTINUED)*

Interventions *(Continued)*

- Consider pacemaker therapy for bradycardia unresponsive to oxygenation, ventilation, and pharmacologic interventions.

- Administer sodium bicarbonate if the child is acidotic.

Rationales *(Continued)*

- To treat bradycardia

- To correct acidosis

OUTCOME:

- The child's cardiac output will be stable.

EVALUATION CRITERIA:

- The child's skin is warm and pink.

- Capillary refill time is normal.

- Heart rate is adequate.

Tachyarrhythmia

Sinus tachycardia is caused by a rate of sinus node discharge that is higher than normal for the age of the patient. This rate may be 140 to 220 beats per minute, depending on the age of the patient.

Supraventricular tachycardia (SVT) occurs when the child has a rapid, regular rhythm, which may be tolerated, particularly in older children, but can lead to cardiovascular collapse, with clinical evidence of shock. SVT may be difficult to distinguish from sinus tachycardia. SVT tends to be a fixed rate and is unresponsive to increases in activity or crying.

Ventricular tachycardia is not commonly found in children, although it may be present in various clinical conditions.

Tachyarrhythmias, which produce cardiovascular instability, should be treated emergently with synchronized cardioversion. Pharmacologic interventions may also be used (such as lidocaine before cardioversion and adenosine for SVT).

NURSING DIAGNOSIS: DECREASED CARDIAC OUTPUT

RELATED TO:

• *Tachyarrhythmia*

Nursing Interventions	Rationales
• Assess the child's cardiac output: - skin color and temperature - strength of peripheral pulses - capillary refill time - level of consciousness.	• To identify signs of decreasing cardiac output
• Assist the child to maintain a position of comfort.	• To promote comfort
• Provide supplemental oxygen, if required.	• To meet increased oxygen demand on myocardial tissue
• Apply a cardiac monitor.	• To provide ongoing rhythm assessment
• Prepare the child for the Valsalva maneuver, if appropriate. Instruct the older child to perform the maneuver independently.	• To facilitate vagal stimulation, causing a decrease in the heart rate
• Establish I.V. access.	• To provide for the administration of adenosine

COLLABORATIVE MANAGEMENT

Interventions	Rationales
• Prepare the infant or child experiencing cardiac collapse for synchronized cardioversion.	• To break re-entry mechanism and establish normal rhythm
• Administer adenosine by rapid I.V. push for the child with SVT.	• To convert rhythm
• Use synchronized cardioversion in a child with cardiovascular instability and clinical evidence of a low cardiac output (0.5–1 J/kg). Repeat cardioversion, if necessary, at 2 J/kg.	• To increase cardiac output

NURSING DIAGNOSIS: DECREASED CARDIAC OUTPUT
(CONTINUED)

COLLABORATIVE MANAGEMENT (CONTINUED)

Interventions (Continued)	Rationales (Continued)
• Administer lidocaine bolus before cardioversion.	• To enhance cardioversion
• Apply infusion therapy with lidocaine.	• To stabilize rhythm
• Administer bretylium if lidocaine is unsuccessful.	• To enhance cardioversion

OUTCOME:	EVALUATION CRITERIA:
• The child will maintain adequate cardiac output.	• The child's skin is warm and pink.
	• Capillary refill time is normal.
	• Peripheral pulses are strong.
	• The child's level of consciousness is normal.

Collapse Rhythms

The collapse rhythms are treated with external chest compression and pharmacologic interventions according to advanced life support steps. Defibrillation may be attempted with ventricular fibrillation.

Asystole is diagnosed in a nonbreathing infant or child by lack of a palpable pulse.

Although ventricular fibrillation is seldom found in infants and children, it is a life-threatening condition that requires cardiopulmonary resuscitation (CPR) and advanced life support procedures. Ventricular fibrillation may be a deterioration of ventricular tachycardia.

NURSING DIAGNOSIS: INADEQUATE TISSUE PERFUSION

RELATED TO:
• *Collapse rhythms*

Nursing Interventions	Rationales
• Assess the child's skin color, temperature, and pulse.	• To provide information about peripheral perfusion
• If you are unable to palpate the pulse, ventilate the patient and perform external chest compressions.	• To provide life support
• Initiate cardiac monitoring.	• To provide ongoing assessment of cardiac rhythm
• Establish I.V. access. Establish intraosseous access for children under 6 years of age.	• To provide a safe and effective route for drug and fluid delivery
• Assist with endotracheal intubation.	• To administer drugs such as epinephrine, atropine, and lidocaine if venous access has not been obtained, to increase or establish a heart rate
• Insert an indwelling urinary catheter and measure urine output.	• To assess renal perfusion

COLLABORATIVE MANAGEMENT

Interventions	Rationales
• Perform CPR and follow pediatric advanced life support protocol for drug therapy.	• To achieve adequate ventilation, oxygenation, and circulation
• Administer I.V. fluids, blood, and plasma, as needed.	• To restore circulating volume
• Assist with defibrillation, if ordered.	• To restore or initiate a spontaneous, organized heartbeat

NURSING DIAGNOSIS: INADEQUATE TISSUE PERFUSION
(CONTINUED)

OUTCOME:
- Adequate tissue perfusion will be restored.

EVALUATION CRITERIA:
- Cardiac rhythm is restored and sustained.

- Urine output remains at 1 mL/kg/hr.

- The child's skin is pink and warm.

- Capillary refill time is normal.

Patient Teaching

Explain the child's condition to the child's parents or caregivers. Use simple, straightforward terms to describe the measures being taken to address the child's condition.

Identify and describe the function of diagnostic, monitoring, and therapeutic equipment.

Documentation

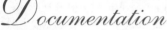

- Cardiac tracing
- Cardiac output, including color, level of consciousness, and peripheral perfusion
- Prescribed medications and patient response
- Defibrillation and cardioversion attempts and patient response

NURSE ALERT:
You may find it helpful to include an actual rhythm strip in the patient's chart with specific interventions noted on the strip.

Defibrillation and Synchronized Cardioversion

Defibrillation is an untimed (asynchronous) depolarization of a crucial mass of myocardial cells that initiates a spontaneous organized beat. In synchronized cardioversion, the principle used is the same as in cardioversion, but the depolarization is timed (synchronous) to avoid the vulnerable phase of the cardiac cycle.

The paddle size for the pediatric patient should be of the largest electrode size to provide good contact over the entire chest area with good separation between the two electrodes. The use of a low-impedance interface medium (electrode gel or cream) is advised.

The electrode paddles are placed so that the heart is situated between them. Although the use of an anteroposterior arrangement, with one electrode on the anterior chest over the heart and the other on the back, is ideal, it is impractical during resuscitation. Therefore, it is recommended that one paddle be placed on the upper right chest below the clavicle and the other, to the left of the left nipple in the anterior axillary line.

The suggested energy dose for defibrillation is an initial dose of 2 J/kg, which should be doubled if defibrillation is unsuccessful. Check the adequacy of ventilation and oxygenation, and make corrections to acidosis before attempting further defibrillation.

Follow the same procedures for synchronized cardioversion, except the dose is 0.5 to 1.0 J/kg. Be sure to activate the synchronizer circuit before administering the dose. Check older models that require the QRS to be upright for proper activation. Discharge buttons must be pressed and held until the countershock is delivered.

NURSE ALERT:
Make sure that no one is in contact with the patient or the bed when defibrillation is attempted.

Overview: Congenital Heart Disease

Human heart development occurs mostly between the 4th and 7th weeks of fetal life, during which developmental errors may result in congenital heart defects. Heart defects occur in about 1% of all live births and are the main cause of death (except for prematurity) among congenital anomalies during the first year of life. Children born with congenital heart disease have a defect in the structure of the heart or in one or more of the large blood vessels leading to or from the heart.

About 90% of congenital heart defects are thought to be due to a combination of genetic and environmental factors.

A few specific maternal diseases, including first-trimester exposure to rubella, insulin-dependent diabetes, and cytomegalovirus, have been implicated in congenital heart disease. Other prenatal or maternal factors that may increase the risk of congenital heart defects include poor nutrition, alcoholism, ingestion of lithium salts, and advanced maternal age.

Children with a family history of congenital heart disease, with Down syndrome or other chromosomal abnormalities, or with other congenital defects are at risk for congenital heart disease. Because of the advances in cardiology today, many more children with severe lesions are surviving beyond the first year of life.

Increasing numbers of infants undergo primary repair of complex congenital heart defects. The infant patient has many needs because of the seriousness of the surgery and the different anatomic, physiologic, and emotional requirements.

Maintaining adequate cardiac output is the major determinant of survival after cardiac surgery. Identifying subtle changes is critical to awareness and prevention of life-threatening complications.

The child must be monitored for distal pulses, temperature of the extremities, skin color, oliguria, altered filling pressures, and low blood pressure to assess the adequacy of cardiac output and to determine if any action should be taken. Arrhythmias are also a postoperative occurrence in response to surgical repair.

CONGENITAL HEART DEFECTS

DEFECT AND PATHOPHYSIOLOGY	ASSESSMENT AND PHYSICAL	PLAN OF CARE FINDINGS
Atrial septal defect A hole in the atrial septum, causing the right side of the heart to take on the added burden caused by a left-to-right shunt	• Symptoms are rare in an infant or a young child • Cardiac enlargement	• Early open heart surgery to close defect

CONGENITAL HEART DEFECTS (*CONTINUED*)

DEFECT AND PATHOPHYSIOLOGY	ASSESSMENT AND PHYSICAL	PLAN OF CARE FINDINGS
Atrial septal defect (*continued*)	• Heart failure, pulmonary hypertension, or atrial arrhythmias may occur in the fourth decade of life • Heart murmur	
Small ventricular septal defect A defect in the ventricular septum, causing increased pressure within the left ventricle to force blood into the right ventricle	• Clinical presentation is related to the size of the defect • Child may range from symptom-free to symptoms of congestive heart failure • Pulmonary hypertension may develop	• Antibiotic prophylaxis if risk of endocarditis • May spontaneously close by 2 years of age
Moderate ventricular septal defect	• Same as for small ventricular septal defect	• Diuretics to reduce hypertension • Surgery usually not required because condition tends to improve spontaneously
Large ventricular septal defect	• Cyanosis in presence of frank pulmonary edema • Signs of heart failure	• Diuretics to reduce edema • Cardiopulmonary bypass required; often surgery is postponed until early childhood or a staged procedure is done in babies

CONGENITAL HEART DEFECTS (*CONTINUED*)

DEFECT AND PATHOPHYSIOLOGY	ASSESSMENT AND PHYSICAL	PLAN OF CARE FINDINGS
Patent ductus arteriosus Oxygenated blood recycles from the aorta to the pulmonary artery through the ductus, causing an overburdening of the pulmonary circulation	Small: • Child may be symptom-free • Dyspnea • Full and bounding pulses on exertion • Growth retardation Large: • Severe heart failure may develop	• Surgical correction; indomethacin to close the ductus
Aortic stenosis Narrowing of the aorta above, below, or at the level of the aortic valve; stenosis worsens as child grows; results in decreased blood flow out of the left ventricle	• Prominent left ventricle • Dyspnea • Exercise intolerance may be present • May produce congestive heart failure if severe	• Balloon valvuloplasty; open aortic valvotomy • Aortic valve replacement is usually delayed until the child stops growing
Pulmonary stenosis Results in decreased blood flow from the right ventricle to the pulmonary artery	• May be asymptomatic or have moderate to severe symptoms • Cyanosis in congestive heart failure in severe cases • Endocarditis	• Cardiac catheterization and balloon valvuloplasty or surgical valvotomy • Antibiotic prophylaxis

CONGENITAL HEART DEFECTS (CONTINUED)

DEFECT AND PATHOPHYSIOLOGY	ASSESSMENT AND PHYSICAL	PLAN OF CARE FINDINGS

Tetralogy of Fallot
 	
Combination of four defects: stenosis or narrowing of the pulmonary artery, hypertrophy of the right ventricle, overriding of the aorta, and ventricular septal defect
	• Cyanosis
	
	• Clubbing of fingers and toes
	
	• Child squats to ease breathing
	
	• Severe dyspnea with exercise
	
	• Cyanotic attacks or spells in infant
	
	• Frequent respiratory infections
	
	• Failure to thrive
		• Staged surgery:
		  - palliative shunt
		  - total correction with cardiopulmonary bypass

Coarctation of the aorta A localized narrowing of the aortic arch or descending aorta; arterial blood bypasses the obstruction to reach the lower part of the body through collateral vessels, which become greatly enlarged	• Normal brachial and radial pulses • Absent or weak delayed femoral pulses • Prominent left ventricle • Left ventricular hypertrophy	• Surgery for all but the mildest cases • Affected section is removed and either anastomosis is performed or a graft is used

CONGENITAL HEART DEFECTS (*CONTINUED*)

DEFECT AND PATHOPHYSIOLOGY	ASSESSMENT AND PHYSICAL	PLAN OF CARE FINDINGS
Transposition of the great arteries Aorta and pulmonary arteries are transposed, resulting in the aorta arising from the right ventricle and the pulmonary artery from the left ventricle; as the ductus arteriosus and foramen ovale begin to close, progressive cyanosis develops; other defects must be present for life to be maintained (without treatment, child is not expected to survive first year of life)	• Child becomes increasingly blue and acidotic • Breathlessness and heart failure are likely to follow • Slightly enlarged heart appears as an egg lying on its side • Echocardiography confirms diagnosis	• Shunt is created between the systemic and pulmonary circuits to allow mixing of blood; prostaglandin E administration and balloon atrial septostomy are used as palliative measures • Corrective surgery is necessary

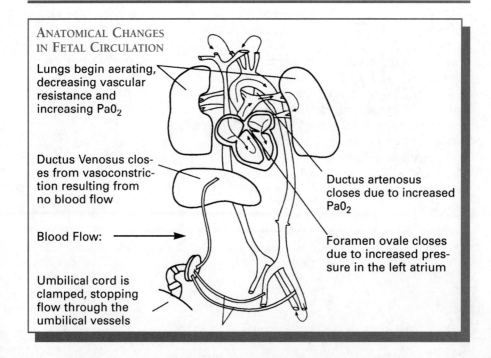

ANATOMICAL CHANGES IN FETAL CIRCULATION

Lungs begin aerating, decreasing vascular resistance and increasing PaO$_2$

Ductus Venosus closes from vasoconstriction resulting from no blood flow

Blood Flow: ⟶

Umbilical cord is clamped, stopping flow through the umbilical vessels

Ductus artenosus closes due to increased PaO$_2$

Foramen ovale closes due to increased pressure in the left atrium

NURSING DIAGNOSIS: INEFFECTIVE FAMILY COPING

RELATED TO:
• *Diagnosis and prognosis of the child with a congenital heart defect*

Nursing Interventions	Rationales
• Explore the family's concerns and feelings of fear, guilt, anger, grief, and inadequacy.	• To establish rapport and reduce anxiety
• Provide information and support to the parents or caregivers. Encourage them to be involved in the child's care.	• To help caregivers comfort the child
• Explain and, if necessary, repeat information and instructions about the child's condition and care.	• To reduce misunderstandings
• Answer the caregivers' questions honestly and allow time for additional questions and information sharing.	• To promote understanding
• Explain diagnostic and therapeutic measures as well as equipment being used.	• To reduce anxiety

COLLABORATIVE MANAGEMENT

Interventions	Rationales
• Consult with other health care providers to help explain the reality of the diagnosis to the caregivers.	• To prevent unrealistic expectations

NURSING DIAGNOSIS: INEFFECTIVE FAMILY COPING *(CONTINUED)*

COLLABORATIVE MANAGEMENT *(CONTINUED)*

Interventions *(Continued)*
- Encourage the parents or other caregivers to contact support groups, clergy, or other resources, as appropriate.

Rationales *(Continued)*
- To establish a support network

NURSE ALERT:
It is important to explore a family's religious beliefs and the role religion plays in the family members' lives. Religious affiliations may have an impact on the family's attitudes regarding death and dying and emergency care, such as blood transfusions.

OUTCOME:
- The family will exhibit adequate coping skills.

EVALUATION CRITERIA:
- The parents or caregivers verbalize feelings, questions, and concerns.

- The parents or caregivers take an active role in the child's care.

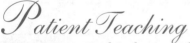
Patient Teaching

Explain basic cardiac anatomy, the child's anatomic defect, and surgical and medical alternatives for correcting the defect or managing its effects. Use simple, direct terms, and models or diagrams, as appropriate.

Identify and explain the function of diagnostic, monitoring, and therapeutic equipment.

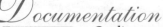
Documentation
- Cardiovascular function, especially arrhythmias or evidence suggestive of congestive heart failure
- Intake and output
- Medications, titration of drips, drug levels of digoxin, and patient response

- Electrolyte values
- Arterial blood gas levels
- Vital signs

Overview: Congestive Heart Failure

Congestive heart failure results from myocardial dysfunction and cardiac output that is inadequate to meet the metabolic demands of the body. In a child, it may be caused by increased cardiac workload, impaired cardiac contractility, an alteration in the order or degree of cardiac contraction, or a combination of these factors.

NURSING DIAGNOSIS: DECREASED CARDIAC OUTPUT

RELATED TO:
- *Myocardial dysfunction*

Nursing Interventions	Rationales
• Assess the child's cardiac output: - skin color and temperature - strength of peripheral pulses - capillary refill time - level of consciousness.	• To identify signs of decreasing cardiac output
• Assist the child to maintain a position of comfort.	• To promote comfort
• Apply a cardiac monitor.	• To provide ongoing rhythm assessment
• Establish I.V. access.	• To provide for the administration of adenosine
• Monitor serum electrolyte levels.	• To identify decreased potassium levels, which may increase the risk of digoxin toxicity
• Limit the child's physical activity and maintain normothermia.	• To decrease metabolic demands, which require increased cardiac output

NURSING DIAGNOSIS: DECREASED CARDIAC OUTPUT
(CONTINUED)

COLLABORATIVE MANAGEMENT

Interventions	Rationales
• Administer digoxin, as ordered. Be sure to monitor for signs of digoxin toxicity.	• To improve the force of ventricular contraction
• Administer angiotensin-converting enzyme inhibitor therapy, as ordered.	• To decrease afterload

OUTCOME:	EVALUATION CRITERIA:
• The child will maintain adequate cardiac output.	• The child's heart rate is strong and within normal limits.
	• Peripheral perfusion is adequate.

NURSING DIAGNOSIS: INEFFECTIVE BREATHING PATTERN
RELATED TO:
• *Pulmonary congestion and edema*

Nursing Interventions	Rationales
• Place the patient in an upright or semi-Fowler's position. Avoid restrictive clothing.	• To improve respiratory excursion
• Monitor the child's: - respiratory rate - work of breathing - pulse oximetry.	• To identify signs of increasing respiratory distress
• Restrict fluids, as ordered.	• To prevent excessive pulmonary edema
• Comfort the child, as appropriate. Encourage the family to comfort the child.	• To reduce anxiety and consequential increased oxygen demands
• Monitor urine output, general edema, jugular vein distention, and daily weight.	• To provide information about fluid retention

COLLABORATIVE MANAGEMENT

Interventions
- Administer supplemental oxygen, as ordered.

- Administer diuretics, as ordered.

Rationales
- To reduce respiratory distress

- To eliminate excessive fluid retention

OUTCOME:
- The child will maintain adequate ventilation.

EVALUATION CRITERIA:
- The child's skin color is normal.

- Respiration is within normal limits.

- The child rests quietly, with little or no sign of respiratory distress.

Patient Teaching

Explain the basic principles of care and equipment to the parents or caregivers.

If the child is to receive drug therapy after discharge, instruct the parents or caregivers about the following:
- Administration technique
- Potential effects of drug toxicity
- Flexibility or lack of flexibility of administration schedule
- When to contact a health care provider

Explain the importance of supplemental potassium requirements when receiving diuretics.

Instruct the parents or caregivers about the dose and schedule for digoxin therapy, if it is ordered for the child. Emphasize that the drug must be dispensed accurately and on a regular schedule. Review the signs of digoxin toxicity.

Documentation

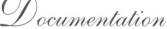

- Cardiovascular and respiratory assessments.
- Cardiac rhythm and any arrhythmia events with treatment and response
- Digoxin levels, electrolyte values, strict intake and output
- Changes in patient status and response to interventions

Nursing Research

A study conducted regarding the identified needs of parents or caregivers of children in the ICU ranked the need for information and knowledge among the most important. Implications of this finding reinforce the idea that parents and caregivers as well as patients are dependent on pediatric nurses.

Fisher, M. D. "Identified Needs of Parents in a Pediatric ICU." *Critical Care Nurse* 14 (June 1994): 82–90.

Chapter 8. Gastrointestinal System

▽ ▽ ▽ ▽ ▽ ▽ ▽

Introduction

SEE TEXT PAGES

Many of the diseases of childhood are associated with some form of vomiting and diarrhea, which puts children at risk for alterations in hydration status. Other GI problems may result in constipation, abdominal pain, or nausea.

Overview: Gastroenteritis

Gastroenteritis, an inflammation of the GI tract, is a common problem that may lead to dehydration if fluids are not replaced.

A child with mild dehydration may be treated with frequent small amounts of clear liquids. A child with moderate or severe dehydration requires immediate infusion of fluids. Specific plans are formulated for the degree and type of dehydration.

CLINICAL SIGNS OF DEHYDRATION

ASSESSMENT FOCUS	5% DEHYDRATION	10% DEHYDRATION
Skin	Loss of turgor	Mottled with poor capillary return
Fontanelle	Mildly depressed	Acutely depressed
Eyes	Sunken	Profoundly sunken
Peripheral pulses	Normal	Weak
Mental state	Listless	Lethargy or coma
Heart rate	Mildly increased	Tachycardia
Mucous membranes	Tacky	Dry

NURSING DIAGNOSIS: FLUID VOLUME DEFICIT

RELATED TO:
- *Vomiting, diarrhea, decreased oral intake*

Nursing Interventions	Rationales
• Assess the presence of nausea, vomiting, or diarrhea, including: - character - frequency.	• To determine the source of fluid loss
• Maintain strict intake and output records.	• To provide accurate information about intake and losses
• Assess urine output for quantity, and measure specific gravity.	• To maintain urine output of no less than 1 mL/kg/hr.
• Assess for elevated temperature, irritability, flaccidity, lack of expression, whiny cry, listlessness, anorexia, and vomiting.	• To identify signs of severe dehydration and shock
• Assess for fluid or weight loss, dry skin and mucous membranes, and decreased serum potassium or sodium levels.	• To identify signs of severe dehydration and shock
• Establish I.V. access for volume replacement.	• To administer I.V. fluids
• Instruct the parents or caregivers to give clear fluids for 24 hours and gradually introduce a normal diet once the child has returned home.	• To maintain hydration at normal levels

COLLABORATIVE MANAGEMENT

Interventions	Rationales
• Administer I.V. therapy: bolus and maintenance fluids.	• To assure adequate hydration
• Administer sodium bicarbonate, as necessary.	• To correct acidosis

COLLABORATIVE MANAGEMENT (CONTINUED)

Interventions (Continued)

- Administer antibiotics if there is a likelihood of systemic spread of bacterial infection.

- Do not treat with antidiarrheal agents.

Rationales (Continued)

- To reduce risk of infection

- To avoid persistence of an abnormal bowel flora

OUTCOME:

- The child's hydration status will return to normal.

EVALUATION CRITERIA:

- The level of consciousness is normal.

- Urine output and capillary refill time are normal.

- Normal acid-base balance is maintained.

- Vomiting and diarrhea are reduced and, eventually, absent.

NURSING DIAGNOSIS: ALTERED NUTRITION (LESS THAN BODY REQUIREMENTS)

RELATED TO:
- *Dietary intake or malabsorption*

Nursing Interventions

- Assess appetite changes:
  - poor or excessive
  - presence of illness
  - diagnosis.

- Assess presence of:
  - nausea
  - vomiting or spitting up
  - diarrhea
  - characteristics of vomitus or diarrhea
  - frequency
  - persistence
  - amount
  - associated conditions of vomiting or stools.

Rationales

- To determine health status and effect of illness

- To gather data about emesis

NURSING DIAGNOSIS: ALTERED NUTRITION (LESS THAN BODY REQUIREMENTS) *(CONTINUED)*

Nursing Interventions *(Continued)*	Rationales *(Continued)*
• Assess the child's height and weight.	• To determine anthropometric data
• Assess abdominal girth, bowel sounds, and distention.	• To perform a complete GI assessment
• Place the child in a comfortable position for feeding and meals.	• To enhance movement of nourishment by gravity and peristalsis and to prevent vomiting or aspiration
• Offer age-appropriate foods of a consistency that does not irritate oral, stomach, or bowel mucosa.	• To promote ingestion and retention of food and to prevent exacerbation of GI disorders
• Maintain nothing-by-mouth status, if prescribed. Offer the infant non-nutritional sucking.	• To provide rest for the GI tract
• Avoid excessive handling of an infant after feeding.	• To prevent possible vomiting from increased stimuli

COLLABORATIVE MANAGEMENT

Interventions	Rationales
• Initiate and monitor I.V. fluid administration.	• To provide short-term fluid and nutritional support

OUTCOME:	EVALUATION CRITERIA:
• The child will maintain adequate nutritional status and fluid volume.	• Daily intake of nutrients is adequate and easily tolerated by the child.
	• There is no evidence of anorexia, nausea, vomiting, diarrhea, bowel distention, or weight loss.
	• The child's weight is normal for his or her height and frame size.

NURSING DIAGNOSIS: DIARRHEA

RELATED TO:

• *Dietary intake, inflammation or irritation of bowel, malabsorption by bowel, ingestion of toxins or contaminants, use of medication or exposure to radiation*

Nursing Interventions

• Assess normal elimination pattern and stool characteristics.

• Obtain stool specimen for laboratory examination in child with diarrhea. Repeat as needed to confirm presence of organisms.

• Place the child on enteric isolation until the diagnosis is confirmed.

• Provide frequent small amounts of fluid and food, gradually increasing amounts as the child's condition improves and he or she is able to tolerate larger amounts of food and fluid.

Rationales

• To acquire baseline information

• To test for toxins, ova or parasites, colonies of infective organisms, occult blood, fat content

• To prevent undue anxiety and transmission of disease in case of bacterial or viral infection

• To allow gradual return to normal diet

COLLABORATIVE MANAGEMENT

Interventions

• Administer and monitor I.V. fluids and electrolytes, as ordered.

• Administer oral rehydration fluids, as ordered.

• Administer anti-infective therapy, antidiarrheals, as ordered.

Rationales

• To allow bowel to rest and to replace lost fluid and electrolytes

• To provide therapy for mild or moderate dehydration

• To destroy or inhibit the growth of microorganisms

OUTCOME:

• The child's bowel patterns will return to normal and adequate nutritional status will be re-established.

EVALUATION CRITERIA:

• Diarrhea is lessened or absent.

• Weight is adequate for the child's height and frame size.

• The child's hydration is adequate.

Patient Teaching

For the child who has experienced fluid volume loss:

Instruct the parents or caregivers to replace fluid losses at the rate of one half cup of rehydration solution for each cup of diarrheal stool.

Explain to the child and his or her caregivers the method of replacing fluids and providing rest for the GI tract.

Provide instructions about oral hydration with small, frequent feedings of ice chips and clear liquids.

Recommend the introduction of a bland diet slowly, as tolerated by the child, after 24 hours of clear fluids.

Identify the signs and symptoms of dehydration and what circumstances necessitate a return to the health care provider.

For the child who has experienced altered nutrition:

Explain to the child and parent or caregiver the method of providing nutrition by I.V. therapy or by nasogastric or gastrostomy tube.

For the child who has experienced diarrhea:

Instruct the child and parents or caregivers in enteric precautions, including hand-washing technique after bowel movement and before eating to avoid transmission or spread of microorganisms that cause diarrhea.

Instruct the child and his or her caregivers how to do the following:
• Reintroduce fluids at room temperature
• Increase feedings of soft foods after fluids are tolerated and stools have decreased
• Gradually continue providing foods as tolerated to resume usual nutritional intake

Explain how to collect a stool specimen and label it properly for laboratory examination.

Tell parents or caregivers to stop using milk or solid foods if diarrhea returns to prevent recurrence of severe diarrhea.

Explain medication administration, if prescribed.

Documentation

- Intake and output
- Bowel movements, including approximate amount and character
- Medications, including those administered by the parents or caregivers, and patient response
- Interventions and patient response
- Vital signs

Overview: Constipation

Constipation is a common problem for children. Parents or caregivers are often concerned about the frequency of a child's bowel movements and any change in the pattern. Constipation is often a minor problem that responds to simple remedies and dietary modification. Some children exhibit severe constipation, which requires more aggressive management.

NURSING DIAGNOSIS: CONSTIPATION

RELATED TO:
- *Inadequate dietary intake and bulk, personal habits, inadequate physical activity, medication, neuromuscular or musculoskeletal impairment, or GI obstructive lesions*

Nursing Interventions	Rationales
• Assess normal elimination pattern and stool characteristics.	• To gather baseline parameters
• Assess abdomen, measure girth, and auscultate for bowel sounds.	• To check for accumulation of stool or reduced peristalsis
• Assess for toilet-training techniques, diet, or environmental changes.	• To uncover reasons for constipation
• Assess for intentional stool withholding and discomfort when defecating.	• To determine reasons the child may be suppressing defecation
• Assess the parents' or caregivers' attitude about bowel habits and toilet training.	• To discover the child's reaction to parents' or caregivers' attitudes that may be causing elimination suppression

NURSING DIAGNOSIS: CONSTIPATION (CONTINUED)

Nursing Interventions (Continued)

- Provide privacy during elimination.

- Allow the child to sit up during bowel elimination.

- Encourage fluid intake and regular activity.

Rationales (Continued)

- To promote elimination

- To provide a normal position for easier bowel elimination

- To enhance bowel motility and prevent hard, dry stool

COLLABORATIVE MANAGEMENT

Interventions

- Add sugar to infant formula. Administer stool softeners, suppositories, or isotonic enema, as ordered.

Rationales

- To promote bowel evacuation when not controlled by fluids and diet

OUTCOME:

- The child's elimination patterns will return to normal.

EVALUATION CRITERIA:

- The child's bowels are evacuated.

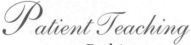

Explain to parents or other caregivers that the change from artificial milk formula or breast milk to cow's milk produces smaller, harder, and less frequent stools that require more effort in passing.

Explain that a child does not have to have bowel elimination every day and that straining is not necessarily a sign of constipation.

Explain how a child may suppress defecation because of bad experiences during toilet training, especially if the child has been punished for accidents.

Instruct parents or caregivers in the dietary inclusion of syrup or corn syrup for an infant and the value of high-fiber foods, such as whole-grain cereals, grains, popcorn, fruit, and vegetables.

Inform parents about food products that tend to be constipating, such as dairy products, rice, apples and apple juice, bananas, and gelatin.

Advise parents or caregivers about the judicious use of stool softeners and the isotonic solution enema when necessary. Use an enema only as directed by a health care provider.

Recommend that the child maintain normal activity levels and instruct the child in abdominal and rectal exercises.

Documentation

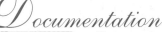

- Characteristics and frequency of bowel movements
- Interventions and patient response

Overview: Appendicitis

Appendicitis results from inflammation of the vermiform appendix, a blind sac situated at the end of the cecum. Although appendicitis is rare in children under age 2 years, it increasingly causes complications and mortality in young children because the appendix frequently perforates before a diagnosis is made.

NURSING DIAGNOSIS: PAIN

RELATED TO:
- *Inflammation of the appendix*

Nursing Interventions	Rationales
• Assess the child's pain, using a pain scale appropriate to the child's age or developmental level.	• To establish a baseline and determine the effectiveness of interventions
• Encourage the parents or caregivers to remain with the child. Provide honest explanations, choices, and preparation for any painful procedures.	• To increase the child's feeling of security
• Make the child as comfortable as possible and respond quickly to complaints of pain.	• To reduce anxiety and provide support

NURSING DIAGNOSIS: PAIN *(CONTINUED)*

Nursing Interventions *(Continued)*
- Demonstrate distraction techniques and other nonpharmacologic pain management techniques.

- Monitor the effectiveness of interventions for pain.

Rationales *(Continued)*
- To help the child cope with pain

- To alter techniques, if necessary

COLLABORATIVE MANAGEMENT

Interventions
- Administer analgesics, as ordered (after diagnosis is made). Be sure to administer pain medication slowly to avoid masking symptoms.

Rationales
- To relieve pain

OUTCOME:
- The child will experience reduced pain.

EVALUATION CRITERIA:
- The child reports a decrease in pain.

- Objective signs of pain, such as facial grimacing and crying, are absent.

- The child uses selected techniques to reduce pain.

NURSING DIAGNOSIS: HIGH RISK FOR FLUID VOLUME DEFICIT

RELATED TO:
- *Nothing-by-mouth status, vomiting, diarrhea, and fever*

Nursing Interventions
- Monitor vital signs, and evaluate the child for signs of dehydration.

- Measure gastric output.

Rationales
- To identify signs of increasing dehydration and to provide early interventions

- To monitor fluid loss

Nursing Interventions *(Continued)*	Rationales *(Continued)*
• Maintain strict intake and output records.	• To determine fluid status

COLLABORATIVE MANAGEMENT

Interventions	Rationales
• Recommend hospital admission for the child with suspected appendicitis.	• To prepare for surgery, if needed
• Administer I.V. fluids, as ordered.	• To maintain adequate hydration
• Insert a nasogastric tube.	• To decompress abdomen

OUTCOME:	EVALUATION CRITERIA:
• The child will maintain adequate fluid volume and will be prepared for surgical procedure, if necessary.	• Urine output is maintained at greater than 1 mL/kg/hr.
	• Urine specific gravity is within normal limits.
	• Fluid and electrolyte intake is adequate.
	• Vital signs are normal.

Patient Teaching

Explain the procedure in terms the child can understand. Encourage the parents or caregivers to help communicate with the child. Keep the parents or caregivers informed.

Documentation

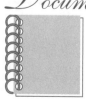

• Objective and subjective pain assessment
• Intake and output
• Nasogastric drainage
• Preoperative laboratory results

Nursing Research

Colic produces stress in about 10% to 20% of infants as well as in their parents or caregivers in the first few months of infancy. Effective interventions for colic include holding and carrying the infant, motion, and, occasionally, a formula change. A randomized, double-blind, placebo-controlled study was conducted to determine the effectiveness of simethicone in infants with colic. The results demonstrated no difference between two populations: one receiving simethicone and one receiving a placebo. Both groups demonstrated "perceived improvements in symptoms," suggesting a placebo effect in both medications.

Metcalf, T. M., et al. "Simethicone in the Treatment of Infant Colic: A Randomized, Placebo Controlled, Multicenter Trial." *Pediatrics* 94 (July 1994): 29–34.

Chapter 9. Reproductive System

▽   ▽   ▽   ▽   ▽   ▽   ▽

Introduction

SEE TEXT PAGES

Interest in body parts, both one's own and those of others, and questions about the body are part of natural curiosity. Children learn and use parental behavior throughout childhood. It is important for children to see parental displays of affection and exchanges of verbal praise. Children also learn attitudes about sexual behavior from the way parents react to public signs of affection.

Young childhood is the ideal time to instruct and promote positive sexual health behaviors. Sexual development is often overlooked or ignored during this time. Health care providers should use opportunities to educate families about sexual development and to promote responsible conduct in sexual matters.

Overview: The Infant or Toddler

The genitals and breasts of the neonate are enlarged in the first few days of life. The vagina may excrete fluids or blood, which may be due to maternal hormonal influences. The toddler begins self-exploration and touches the genitals.

NURSING DIAGNOSIS: KNOWLEDGE DEFICIT

RELATED TO:
• *Age-related concerns about sexual development*

Nursing Interventions	Rationales
• Discuss aspects of sexuality in normal growth and development.	• To provide accurate information to be used as a basis for further discussion
• Provide the parents or caregivers with an opportunity to ask questions.	• To increase the caregivers' knowledge
• Assess parental attitudes regarding affection, if appropriate.	• To determine any areas that require additional explanation or intervention

NURSING DIAGNOSIS: KNOWLEDGE DEFICIT (CONTINUED)

COLLABORATIVE MANAGEMENT

Interventions	Rationales
• Refer the parents or caregivers to other health care providers, as appropriate.	• To provide additional resources

OUTCOME:

• The parents or caregivers will become knowledgeable about sexual development in the infant or toddler.

EVALUATION CRITERIA:

• The parents or caregivers understand correct anatomic terms.

• The parents or caregivers express understanding of the importance of interaction to the physical and emotional health of the child.

Patient Teaching

Explain the anatomy and physiology of the infant's sex organs. Emphasize that some infants may experience breast enlargement or vaginal secretions.

Tell parents or caregivers how the infant learns to recognize affection by affection received.

Explain to parents or caregivers that it is natural for a toddler to be interested in touching the genitals for pleasure and to minimize their reaction to the child's activity. Note that increased masturbation may be a stress-related symptom. Suggest that the parents or caregiver increase the amount of physical affection given to the child.

Advise the parents or caregivers to set limits on the duration of television viewing and to monitor content. Encourage parents or caregivers to talk with their older children about what they have seen on television.

Overview: The Preschool Child

Children become increasingly curious about their own bodies and about the world in general. At this stage, they begin to ask questions about the differences between boys and girls and where babies come from. Short, simple answers that are appropriate to the child's level of comprehension tend to satisfy the child.

NURSING DIAGNOSIS: KNOWLEGE DEFICIT

RELATED TO:
- *Age-related concerns about sexual development*

Nursing Interventions	Rationales
• Discuss aspects of sexuality in normal growth and development.	• To provide accurate information to be used as a basis for further discussion
• Provide the parents or caregivers with an opportunity to ask questions.	• To increase the caregivers' knowledge
• Assess parental attitudes regarding sexuality and the child's sexual exploration and play.	• To determine any areas that require additional explanation or intervention

COLLABORATIVE MANAGEMENT

Interventions	Rationales
• Refer the parents or caregivers to other health care providers, as appropriate.	• To provide additional resources

OUTCOME:	EVALUATION CRITERIA:
• The parents or caregivers will become knowledgeable about the sexual development and activities of the preschool child.	• The parents or caregivers understand correct anatomic terms.
	• The parents or caregivers express understanding of the nature of the child's activities and interest in his or her sexual organs.

Patient Teaching

Tell the parents or caregivers to let the child initiate questions about sexual matters, clarifying information the child is seeking.

Explain that exploratory situations, such as playing doctor, are not motivated by strong sexual desire.

Advise parents or caregivers to set limits for exploratory play and tell the child what are private behaviors.

Address the issue of the Oedipus complex, explaining that this is part of normal development.

Explain the concept of the parent or caregiver as a same-sex role model.

Overview: The School-Age Child

Children's interest in sexual matters decrease when they enter school. During the preadolescent years, they tend to focus on what is happening in their surroundings and in the world in general. Modesty becomes important at this time.

NURSING DIAGNOSIS: KNOWLEDGE DEFICIT

RELATED TO:
• *Age-related concerns about sexual development*

Nursing Interventions	Rationales
• Discuss aspects of sexuality in normal growth and development.	• To provide accurate information to be used as a basis for further discussion
• Provide the parents or caregivers with an opportunity to ask questions.	• To increase the caregivers' knowledge
• Discuss in greater detail, if appropriate, information the child has seen or heard.	• To determine any areas that require additional explanation or intervention

COLLABORATIVE MANAGEMENT

Interventions	Rationales
• Refer the parents or caregivers to other health care providers, as appropriate.	• To provide additional resources

COLLABORATIVE MANAGEMENT (CONTINUED)

Interventions (Continued)

- Collaborate with school health care providers and teachers to provide consistent information to the child.

Rationales (Continued)

- To increase the child's knowledge

OUTCOME:

- The parents or caregivers will become knowledgeable about sexual development and the pre-adolescent's concerns.

EVALUATION CRITERIA:

- The parents or caregivers under-stand correct anatomic terms.

- The child receives accurate infor-mation from parents or caregivers, health care providers, and school personnel.

Patient Teaching

Provide information on upcoming physiologic changes when a child is 9 or 10 years of age.

Use simple language and concrete ideas. Models and illustrations are appropriate for a child this age.

NURSE ALERT:
Education before adolescence may discourage or delay early sexual activity.

Overview: The Adolescent

Puberty heralds the frequently chaotic adolescent years. Sexual feelings and desires emerge and the adolescent undergoes rapid physical, sexual, personal, and intellectual growth. The teenager searches for identity, direction, and a unique place in the world.

Additional concerns at this age include the risk for sexually transmitted diseases, gynecologic infections or conditions, and unwanted pregnancy.

NURSING DIAGNOSIS: KNOWLEDGE DEFICIT

RELATED TO:
• *Age-related concerns about sexual development*

Nursing Interventions	Rationales
• Discuss aspects of sexuality in normal growth and development. Identify any misconceptions and provide accurate information.	• To provide accurate information to be used as a basis for further discussion
• Provide information regarding the physiology of sex, reproduction, sexually transmitted diseases, and pregnancy and contraception.	• To increase patient knowledge and enhance patient safety
• Assess the adolescent's fears, concerns, and perception of the role parents play in sexual development.	• To identify specific areas of concern
• Provide the parents or caregivers with an opportunity to ask questions.	• To increase the caregivers' knowledge
• Provide opportunities to discuss situations in which the adolescent would be required make responsible sexual decisions.	• To determine any areas that require additional explanation or intervention

COLLABORATIVE MANAGEMENT

Interventions	Rationales
• Refer the patient for medical evaluation if sexually transmitted disease or pregnancy is suspected.	• To promote the patient's health and ensure immediate intervention, if needed

OUTCOME:	EVALUATION CRITERIA:
• The parents or caregivers and the patient will become knowledgeable about sexual development and the adolescent's concerns.	• Correct anatomic terms and physiology are understood by parents or caregivers and the patient.

NURSING DIAGNOSIS: KNOWLEDGE DEFICIT (CONTINUED)

OUTCOME:
(CONTINUED)

- The parents or caregivers and the patient will become knowledgeable about sexual development and the adolescent's concerns. (continued)

EVALUATION CRITERIA:
(CONTINUED)

- The patient receives accurate information from parents or caregivers, health care providers, and school personnel.

- The patient is referred for additional medical evaluation, if required.

Patient Teaching

From the adolescent, elicit information about sexual interest, activity, and contraceptive use as well as attitudes and knowledge about sexual matters during routine examinations.

Tell the adolescent you understand that some questions are quite personal, but certain information is important for a complete health history.

Use broadly stated questions, gradually narrowing the focus to avoid appearing threatening.

Facilitate communication between parents or caregivers and the adolescent.

Encourage parents or caregivers to become involved in the adolescent's decisions about responsible sexual behavior.

Assure the adolescent about normal development and that there are many variations among normal physical features.

Inform the adolescent of important normal emotional and psychological changes to be expected.

Provide education on sexuality and sexual behavior, including both physical and psychological aspects.

Explain gender differences in attitude toward sexual relations.

Encourage the adolescent to discuss sex and its place in a relationship before he or she sexually aroused.

Documentation

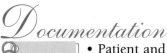

- Patient and parent or caregiver response to education
- Information conveyed, including the use of models or charts
- Information provided for later examination and review by the patient and/or parent or caregiver

Overview: Sexually Transmitted Diseases

Because teenagers are becoming sexually active at earlier ages and in increasing numbers, they commonly become infected with sexually transmitted diseases (STDs), including HIV. In addition, there is a substantial rise in teenage pregnancy.

People younger than age 25 make up two thirds of the estimated 12 million people who acquire an STD each year in the United States, according to the Centers for Disease Control and Prevention. One of every six adolescents—about 2.5 million—becomes infected with an STD every year.

The biology, prevalence, and sequelae are distinct for each STD. Infection with any one STD puts the person at risk for infection with other STDs. Frequently, gonorrhea and a chlamydial infection occur coincidently. See the table below for information on the most prevalent STDs, including assessment and management.

SEXUALLY TRANSMITTED DISEASES

DIAGNOSIS AND ASSESSMENT	MANAGEMENT	NURSING CONSIDERATIONS
Gonorrhea (*Neisseria gonorrhoeae*)	• Penicillin with probenecid	• Identify and treat contacts
Male: Urethritis	• Ceftriaxone or spectinomycin	• Educate about the disease and how it is spread
Female: Postpubertal—cervicitis; prepubertal—vulvovaginitis		• Encourage the use of barrier contraceptives in sexually active teens
		• Assess and treat for chlamydial infection

SEXUALLY TRANSMITTED DISEASES *(CONTINUED)*

DIAGNOSIS AND ASSESSMENT	MANAGEMENT	NURSING CONSIDERATIONS
Chlamydial infection (*Chlamydia trachomatis*) Male: Meatal erythema, tenderness, itching, dysuria, urethral discharge Female: Mucopurulent cervical exudate with erythema, edema, congestion	• Oral tetracycline or doxycycline	• Identify and treat contacts • Educate about the disease and how it is spread • Encourage the use of barrier contraceptives in sexually active teens • Assess and treat for gonorrhea
Syphilis (*Treponema pallidum*) Primary stage: Chancre on penis, vulva, or cervix Secondary stage: Systemic influenza-like symptoms and lymphadenopathy, rash	• Penicillin or doxycycline	• About 95% is transmitted sexually
Pelvic inflammatory disease (PID) Infection of the upper female genital tract (endometrium and fallopian tubes)	• Treat along with underlying infection, usually gonorrhea or chlamydial infection • Oral I.V. antibiotics	• Most commonly caused by an STD, especially gonorrhea or chlamydial infection • Continues to increase among teenagers, although the overall incidence has stabilized or even decreased • Local inflammatory reaction may destroy endothelial tissue; cause tubal scarring and, tubal occlusion; and, ultimately, lead to infertility

SEXUALLY TRANSMITTED DISEASES (CONTINUED)

DIAGNOSIS AND ASSESSMENT	MANAGEMENT	NURSING CONSIDERATIONS
Genital herpes (*Herpesvirus hominis* — type 2) Small, painful vesicles on genital area, buttocks, and thighs	• No known cure; acyclovir lessens healing time and pain	• Can be transmitted to infant during birth
Trichomoniasis (*Trichomonas vaginalis*) Pruritus and edema of external genitalia Foul-smelling, greenish vaginal discharge Sometimes postcoital bleeding	• Oral metronidazole	• Warn patient not to drink alcohol while on medication and for at least 48 hours after last dose
Human papillomavirus Warts on any part of male or female genitalia	• Topical application of podophyllin or trichloroacetic acid • Freezing with liquid nitrogen • Intravaginal and external application of 5-fluorouracil • Laser therapy	• Treat all lesions due to relation to cancer

SEXUALLY TRANSMITTED DISEASES (CONTINUED)

DIAGNOSIS AND ASSESSMENT	MANAGEMENT	NURSING CONSIDERATIONS
Human immunodeficiency virus infection May be asymptomatic to active AIDS Weight loss, night sweats, diarrhea, lymphadenopathy, recurrent infections	• Comprehensive medical management regarding possible drug therapy	• Patients need counseling regarding sexual activity and pregnancy prevention • Provide comprehensive counseling

NURSING DIAGNOSIS: KNOWLEDGE DEFICIT

RELATED TO:
• *Workup, treatment, and prevention of STDs*

Nursing Interventions	Rationales
• Diagnose and treat infections of the lower genital tract promptly.	• To prevent spread to upper genital tract
• Explain transmission, treatment, and prevention of STDs. Identify the relation between STDs and PID as well as certain types of cancer.	• To increase patient knowledge
• Explain the importance of notifying sexual contacts of the infection.	• To prevent disease transmission and reinfection
• Instruct the patient in the use of prescribed medications. Emphasize the importance of completing the entire course of treatment. Stress the importance of returning for follow-up testing.	• To ensure resolution of the infection
• Explain the various diagnostic tests, such as urethral or cervical culture.	• To alleviate patient anxiety about the procedures

NURSING DIAGNOSIS: KNOWLEDGE DEFICIT (*CONTINUED*)

Nursing Interventions *(Continued)*

- Instruct the patient to refrain from sexual activity until the infection has been resolved, if appropriate. Discuss issues related to chronic conditions, such as herpes and AIDS.

- Explain the use of contraception in preventing the transmission of disease.

Rationales *(Continued)*

- To promote effective treatment

- To promote patient safety

COLLABORATIVE MANAGEMENT

Interventions

- Administer antibiotics, as ordered. Note that in severe cases, I.V. medication may be required as well as hospitalization.

NURSE ALERT:
Warn the patient being treated with metronidazole (Flagyl) not to consume alcohol.

- Refer the patient for pregnancy testing, if appropriate.

- Refer the patient for psychological counseling, if appropriate.

Rationales

- To treat bacterial infection

- To begin appropriate interventions

- To address underlying issues causing inappropriate sexual activity and to aid in adjustment to a chronic and potentially fatal condition

NURSING DIAGNOSIS: KNOWLEDGE DEFICIT (CONTINUED)

OUTCOME:

- The patient will understand issues related to STDs, including risk factors and preventive measures.

EVALUATION CRITERIA:

- The patient complies with treatment regimen.

- The patient verbalizes an understanding of the risks, causes, effects, treatment, and outcome of STDs.

- The patient understands his or her responsibility regarding sexual behavior.

Patient Teaching

Educational intervention is vital to reducing the incidence of STDs in adolescents.

Instruct teens to make intelligent, self-directed decisions about their health and to learn how to alter or avoid behavior that puts them at risk for STDs.
- Avoid sexual exposure to an STD or HIV infection.
- Do not use injected drugs or share needles if already using such drugs.
- Resist peer pressure to be involved in high-risk behavior.
- Avoid exposing others when infected.
- Get prompt medical care if infection is suspected.
- Follow and complete treatment.
- Ensure that all sex or drug-use partners get medical care when any one is infected.
- Share accurate information and advice about STDs with peers.
- Be a positive role model.
- Seek the help of others on STD issues.
- Promote STD education.

Documentation

- Sexual and gynecologic history, including the following:
  - Contraceptive method
  - STD prevention methods
  - Number of sexual partners
  - Last menstrual period
- Clinical findings and laboratory test results
- Intervention, education, and patient response

Overview: Teenage Pregnancy

Every year 1 in 10 adolescent girls in the United States becomes pregnant; this is about 1 million girls under the age of 20. More than half of these pregnancies result in a birth. Most teenage mothers are keeping their babies. Consequently, there are 1.3 million babies living with teenage mothers, most of whom are unmarried. These girls and their unborn infants are at high risk for complications, both of pregnancy and of delivery.

Premature labor, low-birth-weight infants, high neonatal mortality, pregnancy-induced hypertension, iron deficiency anemia, fetopelvic disproportion, and prolonged labor are major complications of teenage pregnancies. With quality prenatal care early in the pregnancy, the progress and outcome of these pregnancies improve and are comparable to those of the pregnancies of older women.

NURSING DIAGNOSIS: ALTERED HEALTH MAINTENANCE MANAGEMENT

RELATED TO:
- *Lack of information about pregnancy, contraception, and family planning*

Nursing Interventions	Rationales
• Assess the adolescent's knowledge base regarding the menstrual cycle, sexual activity, and the possibility of pregnancy.	• To determine areas for further discussion and exploration
• Discuss various forms of contraception and the explanations, advantages, and disadvantages of each. Provide written information for later review.	• To provide accurate information for use in decision making

Nursing Interventions *(Continued)*

- Assess the adolescent's support systems, resources, parental involvement in family planning, and sexual health.

- Provide accurate and nonjudgmental information regarding pregnancy options.

- Assess the adolescent's and family's values and religious affiliations.

- Emphasize the need for early prenatal care.

Rationales *(Continued)*

- To encourage the development of a support network

- To increase patient knowledge

- To determine the impact on family planning choices and provide appropriate interventions

- To promote healthier pregnancy

COLLABORATIVE MANAGEMENT

Interventions

- Refer the patient to the appropriate health care provider for prenatal care.

- Provide contraceptives, as prescribed.

Rationales

- To promote the patient's health and safety

- To prevent unplanned pregnancy

OUTCOME:

- The patient will make informed decisions about family planning, contraceptive methods, and sexual activities.

EVALUATION CRITERIA:

- The pregnant adolescent receives information about her condition and situation to enable well-informed decisions.

- The pregnant adolescent receives support for the decisions she makes.

- The sexually active adolescent makes responsible decisions regarding sexual activity, disease prevention measures, and contraceptive methods.

Patient Teaching

Instruct the teenager (and parents or caregivers, when appropriate) about family planning. Provide written materials to reinforce verbal counseling.

Adolescents who have not discussed their sexual practices with their parents often seek the assistance of the nurse in disclosing this information.

Documentation

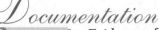

- Evidence of STDs, contraception practices, previous pregnancies, and last normal menstrual period
- Patient and parent or caregiver teaching regarding STDs, pregnancy, counseling, and referrals

Overview: Sexual Assault, Rape, and Abuse

Statistics show that a child is sexually assaulted every 2 minutes in the United States. One of three girls and one of five boys will become a victim of a sexual assault before reaching the age of 18. Although the legal definition of sexual abuse varies by state, most define it as any sexual contact or sexual activity between a child and an adult, whether forcefully, threatened, coerced, bribed, or tricked. There may be no physical symptoms of abuse, but the child may suffer lifetime psychological trauma. Most child sexual abuse offenders are relatives, family friends, or other well-known and trusted adults.

NURSING DIAGNOSIS: HIGH RISK FOR INJURY

RELATED TO:
- *Alleged or suspected sexual abuse*

Nursing Interventions	Rationales
• Establish a rapport with the child and ask open-ended questions.	• To facilitate history taking and encourage the child to discuss aspects of the situation more easily
• Determine the child's fears and concerns early in the interview.	• To reassure the child that he or she has not done anything wrong and has your support
• Refrain from negative facial expressions, body language, or verbal responses.	• To avoid adding to the child's anxiety
• Conduct the examination in a head-to-toe manner.	• To avoid overemphasis of the genitalia or anus and to examine other areas for signs of abuse
• Assist in the collection of specimens for laboratory tests, following protocol for collecting forensic specimens.	• To collect evidence and determine the presence of an STD

COLLABORATIVE MANAGEMENT

Interventions	Rationales
• Report suspected abuse to child protective agencies and the police.	• To help protect the child from further abuse
• Refer the child and family for comprehensive therapy.	• To treat psychological trauma
• Administer treatment for actual or suspected STDs.	• To promote the child's health and resolve any treatable infection

OUTCOME:	EVALUATION CRITERIA:
• The child will be accurately screened for sexual or physical abuse, rape, or STDs and receive appropriate treatment.	• The child receives treatment.
	• Measures are taken to prevent recurrence of the abuse.

Patient Teaching

Parents or caregivers need information about STD screening, examination, treatment, and referrals to child protection agencies.

Alert parents or caregivers to the possibility of regressive behavior.

Advise the family to seek therapy for further psychological and behavioral assessment and counseling.

Documentation

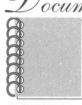

- Details of the interview, including direct quotes from the child
- Laboratory test results
- Forensic specimens collected

Chapter 10. Renal and Urinary System

▽   ▽   ▽   ▽   ▽   ▽   ▽

Introduction

SEE TEXT PAGES

Diseases of the upper and lower urinary tract are common in children. The incidence and type of kidney or urinary tract dysfunction change with the age and maturity of the child. Urinary excretion may be affected by inflammation, damage and scarring of tissue, and dysfunction of the organs or their structures. A deficiency in the kidneys' ability to concentrate urine affects fluid and electrolyte balance.

Overview: Urinary Tract Infection

Between 2% and 3% of girls and less than 1% of boys are at risk for asymptomatic urinary tract infections (UTIs) during childhood. The UTI may involve the urethra, bladder (lower urinary tract), ureters, renal pelvis, calyces, and renal parenchyma (upper urinary tract). Because it is difficult to localize the infection, UTI is the term used to designate the presence of significant numbers of microorganisms in the urinary tract.

NURSING DIAGNOSIS: HIGH RISK FOR INFECTION

RELATED TO:
• *Urinary dysfunction*

Nursing Interventions	Rationales
• Assist in the collection of a urine specimen by way of sterile catheterization technique for culture and analysis.	• To ensure that the specimen is properly collected and to determine the infecting agent
• Explain the test procedures to the child.	• To reduce the child's anxiety
• Advise the parents or caregivers about the use, including dosage and schedule, of any antibacterial drugs prescribed.	• To increase caregiver knowledge and enhance compliance with the treatment regimen

NURSING DIAGNOSIS: HIGH RISK FOR INFECTION (CONTINUED)

Nursing Interventions (Continued)	Rationales (Continued)
• Advise an increase in fluid intake.	• To promote adequate hydration, increase urine output, and prevent urinary stasis

COLLABORATIVE MANAGEMENT

Interventions	Rationales
• Administer antibiotics, as ordered.	• To resolve infection
• Refer the child for additional assessment for functional or anatomic abnormalities, if appropriate.	• To further investigate and treat abnormalities

OUTCOME:
• The child will experience a resolution of the infection and renal function will return to normal.

EVALUATION CRITERIA:
• Laboratory values are within normal ranges.

Patient Teaching

Educate the parents or caregivers about the prevention and treatment of UTI.

Advise the parents or caregivers to teach the child proper hygiene. Explain that, particularly with girls, the child should refrain from prolonged exposure to wet swimsuits and tub bubble baths.

Documentation

• Color and clarity of urine, especially cloudiness, sediment, or foul or strong odor
• Skin integrity in perianal area, especially erythema or rash
• Diagnostic tests
• Patient response to treatment

Overview: Nephrotic Syndrome

Massive proteinuria, hypoalbuminemia, hyperlipemia, and edema point to nephrotic syndrome. It can occur as a primary disease (idiopathic nephrosis, childhood nephrosis, or minimal-change nephrotic syndrome), as a secondary disorder manifesting after or with glomerular damage, or in an inherited congenital form.

NURSING DIAGNOSIS: FLUID VOLUME EXCESS

RELATED TO:
• *Fluid retention and accumulation in tissues*

Nursing Interventions	Rationales
• Assess intake and output. Monitor intake or I.V. infusion carefully.	• To detect fluid accumulation and prevent fluid overload
• Assess changes in edema by measuring abdominal girth and daily weight.	• To identify fluid accumulation
• Measure specific gravity.	• To monitor kidney function
• Use small containers for fluid intake, distributing small amounts throughout the day. Spray the child's mouth with an atomizer. Keep the lips lubricated.	• To limit fluid intake, while preventing thirst and dry mouth and lips
• Monitor vital signs.	• To detect hypovolemia

COLLABORATIVE MANAGEMENT

Interventions	Rationales
• Consult with the dietitian to develop and provide a low-salt diet.	• To prevent fluid retention
• Administer salt-poor albumin, as ordered.	• To prevent intravascular fluid loss and hypovolemic shock
• Administer diuretic therapy, as ordered.	• To provide temporary relief from edema

NURSING DIAGNOSIS: FLUID VOLUME EXCESS (CONTINUED)

OUTCOME:

- The child's fluid status will remain stable.

EVALUATION CRITERIA:

- Intake is restricted to appropriate amounts.

- Excessive fluid retention is detected and treated.

NURSING DIAGNOSIS: HIGH RISK FOR INFECTION

RELATED TO:
- *Lowered body defenses*

Nursing Interventions

- Restrict the child's exposure to infected people.

- Keep the child warm and dry.

- Monitor for early signs of infection.

- Provide skin care, and take care to avoid friction on the skin. Encourage the child to change positions frequently.

Rationales

- To reduce the risk of infection

- To reduce stress and further lower the body's defenses

- To provide an opportunity for prompt intervention

- To prevent skin breakdown and the possibility of introducing infectious agents

COLLABORATIVE MANAGEMENT

Interventions

- Administer antibiotics, as ordered.

Rationales

- To treat infection

OUTCOME:

- The child will be free from infection.

EVALUATION CRITERIA:

- The child's skin is intact, warm, and dry.

- Exposure to other sources of infection is reduced or eliminated.

Patient Teaching

Explain normal kidney function and the pathophysiology of nephrotic syndrome, using age-approriate language for the child.

Stress the importance of restricting fluid intake and maintaining infection control measures.

Documentation

- Intake and output
- Vital signs
- Patient response to diuretic therapy
- Infection prevention measures

Overview: Acute Renal Failure

Although not a common problem, acute renal failure (ARF) is a critical condition in which the kidneys are unable to excrete waste products. Sudden oliguria and electrolyte disturbances are the principal features of ARF. Management priorities are to distinguish whether the cause is prenal, renal, or postrenal and then treat accordingly.

NURSING DIAGNOSIS: FLUID VOLUME EXCESS

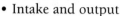

RELATED TO:
- *Decreased urine output of ARF*

Nursing Interventions	Rationales
• Record intake and output every hour.	• To maintain fluid intake at appropriate levels
• Weigh the child daily.	• To assess for fluid retention
• Regulate I.V. therapy and monitor its use carefully.	• To maintain fluid restrictions

• Monitor:
  - vital signs
  - neurologic status
  - electrolyte, ammonia, creatine, and blood urea nitrogen levels.
	• To detect signs of fluid overload, electrolyte imbalance, and monitor renal function

NURSING DIAGNOSIS: FLUID VOLUME EXCESS (CONTINUED)

Nursing Interventions (Continued)	Rationales (Continued)

• Assess for the presence of
  - chest pain
  - dyspnea
  - paradoxical pulse
  - pericardial friction rub
  - narrowing pulse pressure
  - neck vein distention
  - peripheral edema
  - crackles
  - cardiac arrhythmias
  - fever.
	• To detect pericarditis, which may be caused by toxic waste products, as well as pulmonary edema, congestive heart failure, or venous congestion, which may be caused by fluid overload

• Auscultate breath and heart sounds every 2 to 4 hours.	• To detect pulmonary edema and congestive heart failure
• Plan fluid intake to coincide with meals and snacks.	• To limit intake
• Explain fluid restrictions according to the child's understanding.	• To reduce the child's anxiety
• Promote adequate rest and assist the child to maintain a comfortable position.	• To conserve energy and assist in ventilation if pulmonary edema is present
• Prepare the child for dialysis, when necessary.	• To remove waste products and excess fluid

COLLABORATIVE MANAGEMENT

Interventions	Rationales
• Consult with the dietitian to develop and provide a low-salt diet.	• To decrease sodium intake and subsequent fluid retention
• Administer medications, as ordered: antihypertensives, diuretics.	• To regulate abnormalities
• Administer oxygen, as needed.	• To aid gas exchange if pulmonary edema is present

NURSING DIAGNOSIS: FLUID VOLUME EXCESS (CONTINUED)

OUTCOME:

- The child's fluid status will be maintained and cardiac output will be normal.

EVALUATION CRITERIA:

- Serum electrolyte levels are normal.

- The child exhibits no signs of periorbital or peripheral edema, respiratory difficulty, or body weight increase.

- Urine output is regained and maintained.

- The child's intake and output are about equal.

- Fluid restriction is maintained.

- Vital signs are within normal limits.

Patient Teaching

Explain the normal role of kidneys as related to fluid and waste excretion.

Explain the need for fluid restrictions.

Documentation

- Intake and output; hourly I.V. fluids
- Frequent vital signs, daily weights
- Respiratory and cardiovascular assessments

Overview: Enuresis

Enuresis (bedwetting) is not a disease but merely a stage in the child's development.

NURSING DIAGNOSIS: KNOWLEDGE DEFICIT

RELATED TO:
• *Inability to control urination*

Nursing Interventions	Rationales
• Advise the parents or caregivers to have the child take responsibility for wet clothing and bedding.	• To provide reinforcement of the concept that dry clothing and bedding are positive goals
• Reward the child for dry nights.	• To provide positive reinforcement for behavior modification
• Assess the child's urinary elimination patterns.	• To determine normal routines
• Assist in urine specimen collection, as indicated.	• To rule out underlying infection
• Assess parent or caregiver expectations and reactions to incontinence.	• To promote realistic expectations

NURSE ALERT:
The child must be developmentally ready for bladder control. If this is not the case, interventions will not be successful.

• Encourage the child to use the bathroom before bedtime.	• To promote emptying of the bladder and reduce the possibility of nighttime enuresis
• Withhold fluids for a few hours before bedtime.	• To reduce the possibility of nighttime enuresis

COLLABORATIVE MANAGEMENT

Interventions	Rationales
• Use a moisture monitor, provided that the child is sufficiently motivated to respond to the signal.	• To awaken the child at the first sign of moisture and prompt him or her to go to the bathroom
• Administer imipramine, as ordered.	• To decrease urination

OUTCOME:	EVALUATION CRITERIA:
• Episodes of enuresis will be eliminated or reduced.	• The child develops appropriate toileting habits to prevent enuresis.
	• Underlying conditions, if any, are identified and treated.

Patient Teaching

Instruct the parents or caregivers about the safe use of drug therapy, if indicated.

Advise the parents or caregivers that some children take a long time to acquire nighttime continence.

Provide reassurance as needed that the child's enuresis is often within normal limits.

Documentation

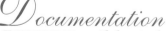

• Abdominal examination findings; may require serial examinations
• Intake and output
• Response to oral and/or I.V. fluid therapy

$\mathcal{C}$hapter 11. Musculoskeletal System

▽   ▽   ▽   ▽   ▽   ▽   ▽

$\mathcal{I}$ntroduction

A child's bones are less resistant to pressure and muscle pull than those of an adult. Consequently, musculoskeletal trauma occurs often in a child. Although a child's bones heal quickly, the functional disruption caused by immobilization while healing results in some physical and emotional alterations in a typically active and curious child.

$\mathcal{O}$verview: $\mathcal{F}$ractures

Pelvic fractures, fractures of the femur, and open fractures require immediate intervention and close monitoring. Pelvic fractures may have associated abdominal and genitourinary injuries. Either complete or incomplete, a fracture line in an extremity may be one of the following:

- Transverse: crosswise, at right angles to the long axis of the bone
- Oblique: slanting but straight, between a horizontal and a perpendicular direction
- Spiral: slanting and circular, twisting around the bone shaft

Types of fractures include:

- Bends—not a complete break
- Buckle or torus—a raised or bulging at the fracture site
- Greenstick—incomplete; does not divide bone
- Complete—a complete division of the bone
- Periosteal hinge—division of the bone; portion of the periosteum remains intact

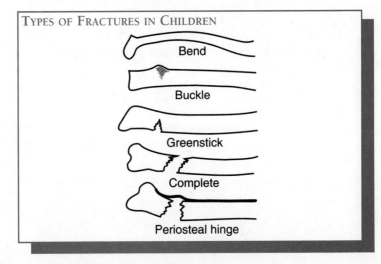

TYPES OF FRACTURES IN CHILDREN

Bend

Buckle

Greenstick

Complete

Periosteal hinge

NURSING DIAGNOSIS: PAIN

RELATED TO:
• *Disability of fracture*

Nursing Interventions	Rationales
• Comfort and reassure the child and his or her parents or care-givers.	• To facilitate further assessment
• Assess: - pain and point of tenderness - pulses distal to fracture site - pallor - paresthesia distal to fracture site - paralysis—movement distal to fracture site.	• To determine the extent of the injury
• Assess the child's level of pain, using an age-appropriate pain scale.	• To determine the need for additional interventions to alleviate pain and to monitor the effectiveness of interventions
• Avoid moving the injured part. Splint or stabilize the joint above and below the injury.	• To prevent pain and reduce the risk of further injury
• Determine the injury mechanism.	• To provide information regarding the type and extent of the injury
• Check for abrasions, cuts, or alterations in the skin surface.	• To identify collateral injuries
• Apply a sterile dressing to open wounds.	• To decrease contamination and reduce the risk of infection
• Reassess neurovascular status.	• To monitor changes secondary to swelling
• Elevate the injured limb.	• To increase venous return
• Apply cold compresses to the injured area.	• To reduce swelling

NURSING DIAGNOSIS: PAIN (CONTINUED)

COLLABORATIVE MANAGEMENT

Interventions

- Administer pain medication, as ordered.

- Administer muscle relaxants, as ordered.

- Assist in manual or surgical reduction, as ordered.

Rationales

- To alleviate or reduce pain

- To reduce muscle strain

- To realign fracture for proper healing

OUTCOME:

- The child's injury will be treated adequately.

EVALUATION CRITERIA:

- The child is free from pain and able to relax.

- The fractured bone is set correctly to facilitate healing.

NURSING DIAGNOSIS: IMPAIRED PHYSICAL MOBILITY

RELATED TO:
- *Musculoskeletal impairment, such as a cast, splint, brace, or bed rest*

Nursing Interventions

- Assess:
  - muscle tone, strength, mass
  - joint mobility, pain, stiffness, swelling
  - movement, activity level.

- Assess bed rest status, activity, and restrictions.

- Avoid restrictions on activity except where specifically ordered.

- Encourage the child to participate in age-appropriate activities.

Rationales

- To acquire data about the child's condition and function

- To determine limits on mobility

- To promote normal mobility

- To provide diversional activities

Nursing Interventions (Continued)	Rationales (Continued)
• Assess other physical effects of immobilization: - elimination - skin breakdown - hypercalcemia - muscle strength loss - contractures - circulatory and pulmonary stasis - anorexia - renal calculi - decreased metabolism and energy - nerve innervation loss.	• To prevent complications
• Provide an opportunity for quiet play and efforts to improve ambulation.	• To promote independence and support efforts to regain and enhance mobility
• Provide, apply, and instruct the child in the use of braces, splints, wheelchair, crutches, and so forth.	• To provide assistance with mobility
• Maintain proper body alignment.	• To promote normal alignment and enhance healing
• Alternate periods of rest with periods of activity.	• To conserve energy
• Assist the child to perform muscle-strengthening exercises.	• To maintain large- and small-muscle strength

COLLABORATIVE MANAGEMENT

Interventions	Rationales
• Administer analgesics before activities, as ordered.	• To promote comfort
• Prepare the child for occupational or physical therapy sessions.	• To facilitate mobility

NURSING DIAGNOSIS: IMPAIRED PHYSICAL MOBILITY
(CONTINUED)

OUTCOME:

- The child will move about appropriately within restrictions imposed by disease or injury.

EVALUATION CRITERIA:

- The child reports that he or she is comfortable and experiencing little or no pain.

- The child participates in age-appropriate diversional activities.

- The child uses any assistive devices correctly.

NURSING DIAGNOSIS: IMPAIRED PHYSICAL MOBILITY

RELATED TO:
- *Skeletal traction*

Nursing Interventions

- Assess the type and purpose of traction.

- Ensure that the components of traction are functional:
  - bandages, frames, and splints are positioned correctly
  - bed is maintained in the correct position
  - patient's body is kept in the correct position
  - tension is constantly applied
  - ropes are taut and knots are secure
  - pulleys are in the proper position and wheels move freely
  - weights are the correct size and hang freely.

- Frequently assess:
  - skin color and temperature
  - pulses and capillary refill
  - numbness and sensation.

Rationales

- To identify the purpose of traction being applied

- To maintain correct traction

- To identify neurovascular changes caused by the traction

Nursing Interventions (Continued)

- Assess pressure points.

- Perform range-of-motion exercises to unaffected joints.

- Clean and dress pin sites. Apply antiseptic ointment. Monitor for signs of infection.

- Assist the child in performing activities of daily living.

- Provide diversional activities as appropriate.

- Encourage the child's family and friends to visit.

Rationales (Continued)

- To prevent skin breakdown

- To prevent contractures

- To reduce the risk of pin site infection

- To promote independence

- To promote activity within the limitations imposed by traction

- To increase social interaction

COLLABORATIVE MANAGEMENT

Interventions

- Administer antibiotics, as ordered.

- Prepare the child for physical or occupational therapy, as appropriate.

Rationales

- To reduce pin site infection

- To promote mobility

OUTCOME:

- The child will maintain an appropriate level of mobility, considering the limitation imposed by traction.

EVALUATION CRITERIA:

- Correct levels of traction are maintained.

- The child shows no signs of complications related to immobility, such as skin breakdown.

Patient Teaching

Inform the parents or caregivers and the child about the hazards of immobility and the importance of medical and exercise regimen compliance. Explain the actual limitation imposed by mobility devices or traction equipment.

Instruct the parents or caregivers and the child in the use of mobility devices, aids, or traction equipment.

Identify environmental modifications that are needed to ensure patient safety, such as removing small area rugs and relocating furniture to improve access to key areas.

Explain and demonstrate activities to improve large-muscle strength and range-of-motion exercises. Suggest activities to prevent boredom while the child is immobilized.

Outline the expected progress in ambulation. Stress the importance of therapy and follow-up.

Documentation

- Assessment of fracture, tissue integrity, and neurovascular status
- Pain assessment, including interventions and patient response
- Patient progress in increasing mobility and in the use of mobility aids

NURSE ALERT:
Documenting neurovascular activity may be accomplished by the use of a neurovascular flowsheet.

Overview: Congenital Hip Dysplasia

Congenital hip dysplasia (CHD) describes inadequate development of the hip, which can affect the femoral head, the acetabulum, or both. The most common congenital defect, CHD is apparent at birth, has various degrees of deformity, and is thought to be due to genetic factors. Both hips are involved in one fourth of the cases; when only one hip is involved, it is usually the left hip. CHD often accompanies other conditions, such as spina bifida.

NURSING DIAGNOSIS: KNOWLEDGE DEFICIT

RELATED TO:
- *Treatment and care of CHD*

Nursing Interventions

- Maintain a harness device or cast. Explain its purpose to the child, if appropriate, and the parents or caregivers.

- Instruct the parents or caregivers in the use of the reduction device.

- Provide skin care while the child is using the cast. Identify measures the parents or caregivers can take to ease skin discomfort.

- Explain and demonstrate range-of-motion exercises to be used once the cast is removed.

Rationales

- To ensure uninterrupted therapy

- To ensure uninterrupted therapy once the child has returned home

- To prevent skin breakdown

- To help restore movement

COLLABORATIVE MANAGEMENT

Interventions

- Explain the treatment that might be used by other health care providers, as appropriate for the child's age:
- Neonate to 6 months: Hip joint is maintained by splinting with harness device.

- Six to 18 months: Gradual reduction with cast immobilization is used. Open reduction may be necessary with a postoperative spica cast.

- Older child: The condition is more difficult to treat and may require operative reduction with preoperative traction, tenotomy of contracted muscles, and any of a number of innominate osteotomy procedures.

Rationales

- To stabilize hip

NURSING DIAGNOSIS: KNOWLEDGE DEFICIT *(CONTINUED)*

OUTCOME:
- Parents or caregivers will be informed regarding the defect and the treatment regimen.

EVALUATION CRITERIA:
- The child's hip remains in the desired position.

- The corrective device is positioned accurately.

- The child's skin is free of irritation and circulation is not impaired.

- The family adjusts its nurturing activities to accommodate the corrective device.

Patient Teaching

Explain physical assessment findings, basic anatomy, pathophysiology of CHD, and treatment regimen.

Emphasize the need to retain the harness device in place at all times.

Explain and demonstrate care techniques, such as bathing, skin care, and range-of-motion exercises, done with the harness or cast in place.

Documentation

- Patient and parent or caregiver response to instruction; when possible, elicit a return demonstration
- Skin integrity
- Neurovascular assessment

Overview: Scoliosis

An abnormal lateral curvature of the spine, scoliosis sometimes has secondary compensatory curves and rotation of vertebral bodies, hyperlordosis (extreme swayback), or kyphosis (pronounced convexity of the upper back). Many girls have some degree of scoliosis that causes little difficulty.

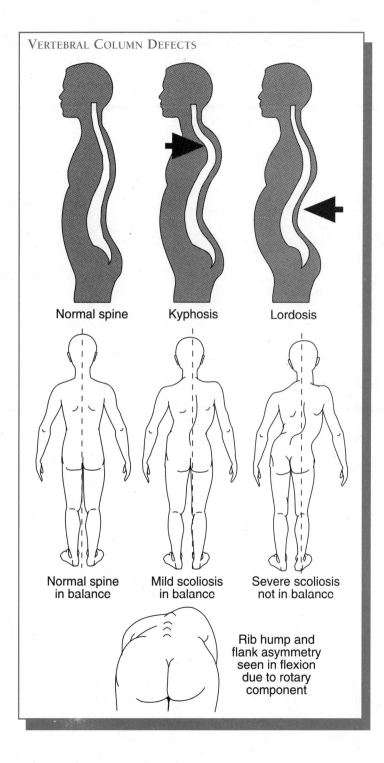

VERTEBRAL COLUMN DEFECTS

Normal spine Kyphosis Lordosis

Normal spine
in balance

Mild scoliosis
in balance

Severe scoliosis
not in balance

Rib hump and
flank asymmetry
seen in flexion
due to rotary
component

NURSING DIAGNOSES: INEFFECTIVE INDIVIDUAL COPING NONCOMPLIANCE

RELATED TO:
- *Developmental age, altered body image, chronicity, and treatment complexity*

Nursing Interventions	Rationales
• Demonstrate and explain the orthotic device and treatment regimens.	• To introduce the device and its use
• Show illustrations of other children wearing the devices as they participate in various activities.	• To help the child identify with others who use the devices
• Stress the importance of careful and frequent monitoring.	• To evaluate progress of the treatment
• Provide realistic decision-making opportunities for the child, such as the selection of flattering clothing.	• To promote the child's feeling of control and encourage participation in the treatment regimen
• Encourage the child to explore his or her feelings about the device.	• To promote communication and understanding of the need for the device
• Encourage the child's family and friends to visit frequently and to engage in social activities.	• To divert the child from the discomfort and anxiety related to treatment
• Emphasize the importance of the child's completing as many activities of daily living as possible.	• To promote independence
• Demonstrate and encourage the child to perform daily supplemental exercises.	• To prevent abdominal or spinal atrophy

COLLABORATIVE MANAGEMENT

Interventions	Rationales
• Refer the child and parents or caregivers for evaluation, if surgical correction is indicated.	• To explore surgical alternatives

COLLABORATIVE MANAGEMENT (CONTINUED)

Interventions (Continued)

• Encourage the child and family to contact support groups, as appropriate.

Rationales (Continued)

• To develop a support network

OUTCOME:

• The child will accept treatment and display adaptation to the changes required by the treatment regimen.

EVALUATION CRITERIA:

• The child maintains normal contact and interaction with family and friends.

• The child completes appropriate self-care requirements.

• The child expresses satisfaction with his or her participation in the care regimen.

Patient Teaching

Teach the child correct posture.

Emphasize that the brace or jacket must be worn constantly, with a 30-minute break in the morning and evening for exercise and general hygiene.

Demonstrate how to check the brace for proper fit and massage pressure areas. Massage should be done at least twice daily.

Demonstrate abdominal and back exercises that will strengthen muscles and improve posture.

Documentation

• Patient response to treatment and instruction
• Degree of spinal curvature
• Postural abnormalities
• General appearance

Overview: Skeletal Trauma from Child Abuse

Child abuse frequently results in injuries that involve the skeletal system. Nurses are legally responsible to report situations in which abuse is suspected: reporting, documenting factual data, acting as an advocate, and focusing on prevention are key nursing responsibilities. It is important for the nurse to keep in mind that abuse occurs across social, ethnic, and economic subcultures.

Child abuse or neglect is defined as harm to a child by a caretaker that is either emotional or physical in nature. The major types of abuse are neglect and physical, emotional, and sexual abuse. See the table below for details on these types and Chapter 10 for in-depth information on sexual abuse.

TYPES OF CHILD ABUSE

TYPE	DEFINITION AND FEATURES
Physical	Nonaccidental trauma - bruises - burns - fractures - other signs of physical harm
Sexual	Assault by an adult, an older child, or a teen for his or her gratification. Activity may range from nontouching gestures to a violent sexual act.
Emotional	Abnormal caregiving behavior or unusual punishment that damages the child's psychological well-being
Neglect	Failure by parents or caretaker to provide basic needs of clothing, food, shelter, education, and medical care to child

NURSING DIAGNOSIS: HIGH RISK FOR INJURY

RELATED TO:
• *Known or suspected child abuse*

Nursing Interventions	Rationales
• Assess and treat the child's immediate injuries.	• To ensure patient safety
• Report suspicions of abuse to social service agency or the police. Make a notation of the report on the child's medical record.	• To ensure patient safety and comply with state statutes
• Document: - child's name, address, telephone number - full names of mother and father or legal guardian - your name and telephone number.	• To record information reported
• Inform the appropriate supervisor or administrative personnel of the report.	• To ensure follow-through for legal requirements
• Provide reassurance and support to the child.	• To allay fears, begin building a trust relationship with the child, and provide some degree of control over the situation
• Inform the parents or caregivers of your report.	• To emphasize that you are concerned about the welfare of the child and to inform them of your legal obligations in reporting suspected child abuse

NURSING DIAGNOSIS: HIGH RISK FOR INJURY (CONTINUED)

COLLABORATIVE MANAGEMENT

Interventions	Rationales
• Refer the family to appropriate counseling or support groups.	• To address the need for interventions for the whole family

OUTCOME:	EVALUATION CRITERIA:
• The child will receive treatment for the chief complaint and will be protected from further abuse or neglect.	• The child's injuries are treated and have begun to heal.
	• The report of suspected child abuse has been filed with the appropriate authorities.
	• The family begins counseling for abuse-related issues.

Patient Teaching

Explain the importance of bonding with child. Help the parent or caregivers learn how to deal with various phases of the child's growth and development. Discuss their expectations for the child's behavior.

Teach parents modeling behaviors.

Clarify the family's understanding of follow-up care.

Recommend support sources, such as crisis nurseries, mental health centers, parenting classes, and hot lines.

Documentation

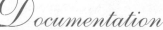

• Accurate documentation of statements by parents or caretakers, including a comparison of statements made to various health care providers
• Assessment findings with particular attention to types, character, and pattern of injuries

NURSE ALERT:
Note that frequent changes in history may point to avoidance of the real cause of the child's injuries.

Chapter 12. Neurologic System

▽   ▽   ▽   ▽   ▽   ▽   ▽

Introduction

SEE TEXT PAGES

Head trauma is the most frequent cause of a neurologic problem in children. Seizures, obstructive problems, brain tumors, congenital vascular malformations, and infectious processes, such as meningitis and sepsis, may also result in neurologic difficulties.

Overview: Head Injuries

Traumatic head injury, a significant, often preventable cause of death and disability in children and adolescents, is sustained by 200,000 children annually in the United States. Most (89%) of those injuries are caused by falls and by bicycle, vehicular, and sporting accidents. A child who survives serious brain trauma is at risk for substantial and sometimes lifelong residual problems.

Head injuries may result from a severe direct blow or indirectly from a sudden jolt (acceleration-deceleration) of the head. Injuries include skull fractures, concussions, cerebral contusions, lacerations, cerebral edema, and hemorrhage.

NURSING DIAGNOSIS: HIGH RISK FOR INJURY

RELATED TO:
• *History of head trauma*

Nursing Interventions	Rationales
• Describe the child's behavior clearly and comprehensively.	• To provide an accurate understanding of the child's condition
• Assess the child's: - gag, swallow, and deep tendon reflexes - ability to speak.	• To ensure that the child's reflexes are adequate to protect his or her airway
• Elevate the head of the bed 15 to 30 degrees.	• To promote cerebral venous drainage

NURSING DIAGNOSIS: HIGH RISK FOR INJURY (CONTINUED)

Nursing Interventions (Continued)	Rationales (Continued)
• Monitor intake and output. Restrict the child's fluid intake in the absence of hypovolemic shock.	• To decrease circulating blood volume to the brain
• Protect the child from injuring himself or herself with restless movements or seizures by padding the side rails, keeping the rails up, and frequent monitoring. Assess, report, and correct other causes of restlessness.	• To prevent additional injury
• Encourage a family member or close friend to be present when the child regains consciousness.	• To relieve anxiety and calm the child
• Avoid the use of sedatives, when possible.	• To prevent respiratory depression and masking of neurologic changes
• Monitor any medications, physical movement, or conditions that may adversely affect the child or treatment outcome.	• To identify potential problems and provide early intervention

COLLABORATIVE MANAGEMENT

Interventions	Rationales
• Schedule appropriate diagnostic testing.	• To evaluate injuries
• Apply a cervical collar, as ordered, being careful not to flex the child's neck.	• To prevent additional injury

NURSE ALERT:
The collar may be removed only after spinal injury has been ruled out.

NURSING DIAGNOSIS: HIGH RISK FOR INJURY (CONTINUED)

OUTCOME:
- The child will be thoroughly assessed for head trauma and will receive appropriate treatment.

EVALUATION CRITERIA:
- The child's head and neck are immobilized until spinal injury is ruled out.

- Injuries are accurately assessed and interventions are begun.

Patient Teaching

Identify important signs relating to the child's level of consciousness that should be observed. Emphasize that changes in the child's level of consciousness are the most important signs to be reported to the health care provider. Instruct the parents or caregivers to awaken the child every 2 hours for the first 24 hours after the injury to assess level of consciousness. Signs to report include the following:
- Seizures
- Changes in consciousness level
- Persistent vomiting
- Unequal pupils
- Weakness or loss of use of extremities
- Slurred speech
- Blurred vision
- Severe headache
- Unsteady gait

Explain to the parents or caregivers that severe headache, restlessness, and agitation should be noted. Acetaminophen may be used to alleviate pain. A bland diet should be provided for the first 24 hours after the injury.

Tell the parents or caregivers that vomiting commonly occurs in even mild head injury but to call the health care provider if it is forceful or persistent.

Documentation

- Primary assessment record
- Historical data, including cause of injury
- Vital signs
- Ongoing neurologic evaluation records
- Medical and nursing interventions, including patient response

- Condition on discharge and admission
- Discharge instructions; possible food or drug interactions with anticonvulsants, if prescribed
- Follow-up care

Overview: Increased Intracranial Pressure

Intracranial pressure (ICP) is above-normal pressure of cerebrospinal fluid (CSF). It can increase acutely, causing neurologic function to rapidly decline, or it can develop slowly, with headache as the only symptom for several weeks until other focal neurologic symptoms appear.

Most of the cases of increased ICP are the result of massive lesions, brain edema, increased CSF volume, increased CSF pressure, or increased blood volume.

NURSING DIAGNOSIS: HIGH RISK FOR INJURY

RELATED TO:
- *Increase in brain tissue, intracranial blood volume, or CSF volume*

Nursing Interventions	Rationales
• Monitor the child's neurologic status every 1 to 2 hours. Sometimes this may be required every 15 minutes.	• To identify changes that may indicate increasing ICP
• Monitor vital signs every 15 minutes to once every hour.	• To identify changes that indicate increased ICP
• Monitor intake, output, electrolyte levels, and urine specific gravity.	• To detect indications of diabetes insipidus
• Elevate the head of the bed and align the child's head and neck.	• To maintain venous flow from the brain
• Describe and record the child's behavior.	• To identify signs of agitation and confusion
• Instruct the older child to refrain from certain activities, such as coughing and straining for bowel movement.	• To prevent an increase in ICP

Nursing Interventions (Continued)

- Encourage the parents or care-givers to comfort the child as much as possible to prevent crying.

- Use restraints only when essential. Check the child frequently if he or she is restrained.

- Schedule nursing activities to avoid tiring the child. Reduce environmental stimuli.

- Follow strict infection control precautions.

- Drain intraventricular catheter device.

- Record ICPs as well as the amount and character of CSF, and maintain proper height alignment.

Rationales (Continued)

- To prevent an increase in ICP

- To prevent unnecessary motion and agitation

- To promote periods of uninter-rupted rest

- To reduce the risk of infection

- To drain excessive CSF

- To detect an increase in ICP

COLLABORATIVE MANAGEMENT

Interventions

- Limit fluids, as prescribed.

- Use dehydration and ventilation to control cerebral blood volume.

- Administer anticonvulsants and mild sedatives, as ordered.

- Shunt tap to remove excess CSF.

- Administer steroids and diuretics, as ordered.

Rationales

- To prevent cerebral edema

- To maintain mean arterial and cerebral perfusion pressures

- To treat adverse effects

- To relieve pressure

- To decrease swelling and fluid retention

OUTCOME:

- The child's condition will stabilize and begin to improve.

EVALUATION CRITERIA:

- The child has an ICP of 0 to 15 mm Hg and cerebral perfusion pressure <50 mm Hg.

- The child's neurologic status is maintained and improves.

NURSING DIAGNOSIS: INEFFECTIVE BREATHING PATTERN

RELATED TO:
• *Increased ICP and alteration in level of consciousness*

Nursing Interventions	Rationales
• Maintain airway patency.	• To ensure effective breathing
• Suction the oropharynx with care.	• To maintain patency without elevating ICP
• Monitor respiratory rate, rhythm, and depth every 15 minutes to once every hour.	• To identify signs of increasing ICP
• Monitor arterial blood gas levels.	• To ensure adequate oxygenation and ventilation

COLLABORATIVE MANAGEMENT

Interventions	Rationales
• Assist with immediate intubation and hyperventilation if the child continues to experience neurologic decompensation.	• To maintain a patent airway and lower ICP
• Hyperventilate the child to maintain $Paco_2$ in the 25-30 mm Hg range (normal 35-45 mm Hg).	• To reduce ICP caused by vasodilation related to elevated $Paco_2$ levels
• Administer paralytics and sedatives, as ordered, for the child who is mechanically ventilated.	• To facilitate the ventilation process

OUTCOME:
• The child will maintain adequate ventilation.

EVALUATION CRITERIA:
• Arterial blood gas levels are within normal ranges.

• Breath sounds are clear.

• The airway remains patent.

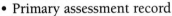

Patient Teaching

Advise parents or caregivers to report signs of increased ICP, such as seizures, changes in the child's level of consciousness, and vomiting.

Explain the equipment used to diagnose, treat, and monitor the child's condition. Explain the procedures the child will undergo.

Describe the effects of medications prescribed for the child, such as sedatives, anticonvulsants, and diuretics.

Documentation

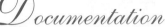

- Primary assessment record
- Historical data, including cause of injury
- Vital signs
- Glasgow Coma Scale ratings
- Arterial blood gas levels
- Intake and output
- Ongoing neurologic evaluation records
- Medical and nursing interventions, including patient response
- Condition on discharge and admission
- Discharge instructions; possible food or drug interactions with anticonvulsants, if prescribed
- Follow-up care

Overview: Status Epilepticus

Although many children may have seizures caused by fever or disease, few progress to the repetitive episodes that point to epilepsy. Status epilepticus is any seizure, single or repeated, that lasts 30 minutes or longer or repeated seizures that have no recovery in between. Seizures are classified as *partial*—a focal motor seizure—and *generalized*—tonic-clonic, typical absence, and atypical absence seizures. Prompt intervention is critical to reducing morbidity and mortality, which are related to seizure duration.

Some syndromes or phenomena may mimic seizures and need to be considered in the differential diagnosis. They include the following:
- Episodes of daydreaming
- Familial chin trembling
- Some migraine headaches
- Breath-holding
- Positional vertigo or syncope

- Shuddering spells
- Psychogenic seizures

NURSE ALERT:
In an actual seizure disorder, the child's seizures proceed in the same manner, whereas psychogenic seizures differ from episode to episode.

NURSING DIAGNOSIS: ALTERED CEREBRAL TISSUE PERFUSION

RELATED TO:
- *Decreased oxygen and glucose supply to the brain*

Nursing Interventions	Rationales
• Secure I.V. access.	• To provide access for medication
• Monitor respiratory effort and assist with ventilation, as needed.	• To promote adequate ventilation
• Turn the child on his or her side.	• To secure airway and facilitate suction of secretions
• Lower the child to the ground or pad the side rails.	• To reduce the risk of injury
• Apply a pulse oximeter.	• To monitor oxygen saturation

COLLABORATIVE MANAGEMENT

Interventions	Rationales
• Administer supplemental oxygen, as ordered.	• To ensure adequate oxygenation
• Administer medications, as ordered. Monitor carefully for adverse effects, such as respiratory depression and hypotension.	• To halt seizure activity and prevent recurrence

OUTCOME:	EVALUATION CRITERIA:
• The patient will maintain adequate oxygenation.	• The child's airway remains patent.
	• Ventilation is adequate.
	• The child's seizure activity is halted.

Patient Teaching

Instruct the parents or caregivers to place the child on the floor and call for emergency services. Remove any immediate environmental hazards.

Explain follow-up evaluation with the neurologist, as indicated.

Overview: Meningitis

Meningitis is an acute inflammation of the meninges. It occurs more commonly in children than in adults, frequently causing death and disability. It is seen most often in children between 1 month and 5 years of age.

NURSING DIAGNOSIS: HIGH RISK FOR INFECTION

RELATED TO:
- *Bacterial invasion of the meninges*

Nursing Interventions	Rationales
• Monitor the child for signs of septic shock.	• To prevent septic shock
• Provide isolation if indicated (usually for the first 24 hours after antibiotic therapy is started).	• To prevent the spread of the disease
• Monitor for signs of: - increased ICP - fever.	• To prevent additional complications
• Decrease environmental stimuli.	• To limit agitation
• Keep the lights off.	• To decrease the effects of photophobia
• Secure I.V. access.	• To administer systemic antibiotics

NURSING DIAGNOSIS: HIGH RISK FOR INFECTION (CONTINUED)

COLLABORATIVE MANAGEMENT

Interventions	Rationales
• Provide airway, ventilation, and circulation support.	• To maintain vital functions
• Administer antibiotics, as ordered.	• To resolve infection
• Administer antipyretics, as ordered.	• To reduce fever

OUTCOME:
• The child will experience a resolution or reduction in infection.

EVALUATION CRITERIA:
• Vital signs are normal.

Patient Teaching

Explain all tests and procedures to parents or caregivers.

Review the medications the child will be taking and the treatments being prescribed for the child.

Emphasize the importance of follow-up examinations once the child has returned home to ensure a return to baseline functioning.

Documentation

- Frequent neurologic assessments, including level of consciousness, motor and sensory activity, orientation, and pupillary response
- Seizure activity; be sure to note the duration, anticonvulsant therapy given, and response to therapy
- Intake and output
- Amount and character of CSF

Chapter 13. Skin and Lymph System

▽   ▽   ▽   ▽   ▽   ▽   ▽

Introduction

SEE TEXT PAGES

Skin is important because of its protective factors: it guards the body from physical, chemical, and biologic abuse; helps control body temperature; and is an effective barrier to the passage of substances in or out of the body.

Overview: Rash

Infants develop diaper dermatitis; many young children develop allergic reactions to environmental factors and are susceptible to parasitic infections. Acne is a common problem among teenagers.

COMMON CHILDHOOD SKIN PROBLEMS

CONDITION	SIGNS AND SYMPTOMS	TREATMENT
Diaper dermatitis	• Irritation of skin, primarily around convex surfaces and skin folds	• Keep skin clean and dry. • Avoid overwashing with harsh soaps. • Change diapers frequently. • Use superabsorbent diapers. • Expose skin to air when possible. • Apply ointments, as directed. • Antifungal or glucocorticoid ointments may be necessary.

COMMON CHILDHOOD SKIN PROBLEMS (*CONTINUED*)

CONDITION	SIGNS AND SYMPTOMS	TREATMENT
Seborrhea	• Distinctive erythematous, scaly eruption • Cradle cap when scalp is involved • Appears in the 2nd or 3rd month of life • May spread rapidly with psoriasis-like lesions covering most of the body • Child is not ill or distressed	• Bathe infant frequently with medicated soap. • Apply mild corticosteroid, as directed. • Loosened scales can be gently brushed away with a soft brush.
Eczema	• Red antecubital spaces, often spreading to the trunk and inguinal creases • May appear on wrists, knee creases, ankles • Causes itching • Scratching frequently may cause secondary staphylococcal infection • Associated with a hereditary allergic tendency	• Minimize bathing. • Use only mild soap when necessary. • Apply topical steroids, as directed. • Apply an emollient cream. • Alter diet to eliminate environmental allergens. • Administer oral antihistamines, as ordered.

COMMON CHILDHOOD SKIN PROBLEMS (CONTINUED)

CONDITION	SIGNS AND SYMPTOMS	TREATMENT
Impetigo	• Highly contagious superficial skin infection • Golden brown crust	• Apply a topical antibiotic, as ordered. • Use systemic antibiotics for extensive lesions. • Wash hands thoroughly after applying topical medication.
Herpes simplex	• Gingivostomatitis—blister-like lesions on the oral mucous membranes • Fever • Irritability • Difficulty swallowing	• Ensure adequate fluid intake. • Apply idoxuridine paint. • Avoid acidic juices. • Offer soft foods.
Scabies	• May be nonspecific finely papular, sparse, highly pruritic rash • May have typical burrow pattern on skin surface	• Apply benzyl benzoate emulsion to skin surfaces below the neck. • All contacts should be treated. • All linens and clothing should be hot-laundered.
Pediculosis capitis (head lice)	• Persistent itch • Secondary dermatitis, papules • White eggs (nits) visible on hair shaft	• Apply 0.5% malathion, permethrim, lindane. • Wash infected objects (combs, hats) with hot soapy water. • Use a nit comb to loosen nits from hair shafts.

COMMON CHILDHOOD SKIN PROBLEMS (CONTINUED)

CONDITION	SIGNS AND SYMPTOMS	TREATMENT
Tinea corporis (ringworm)	• Fungal infection, usually from family pet • Distinctive red, round, scaly patches with some clearing in the center	• Administer topical or oral antifungal agent.
Roseola	• Light pink rash • Follows 3 to 4 days of fever • Not pruritic	• Treat fever with acetaminophen, not aspirin.

Patient Teaching

Instruct the parents or caregivers about medication administration.

Explain the preparation and use of soaks and baths.

Explain the transmission and prevention of contagious infections.

Documentation

• Location, type, and pattern of lesions
• Exudate or erthyema surrounding lesions
• Patient response to interventions

Overview: Acne
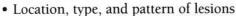

Acne is nearly a universal problem for adolescents; about 70% of the teenage population suffers from its effects. It involves anatomic, physiologic, biochemical, genetic, immunologic, and psychological aspects of some import.

The cause of acne is not clear; however, factors such as emotional stress and premenstrual period in females are related to its development.

NURSING DIAGNOSIS: IMPAIRED SKIN INTEGRITY

RELATED TO:
• *Acne lesions*

Nursing Interventions	Rationales
• Recommend gentle cleaning twice daily.	• To ensure clean skin and to remove comedones and excess oil from sebaceous gland activity
• Promote adequate rest, emotional stress reduction, good nutrition, and fluid intake.	• To promote general health, which may improve skin condition
• Discourage picking or popping of lesions.	• To reduce the risk of infection and scarring
• Encourage the use of water-based cosmetics only. Emphasize that cosmetics must be removed from the face at night.	• To keep pores clean
• Suggest frequent shampooing and a hair style in which the hair is kept off the face.	• To limit contact of oily hair with skin

COLLABORATIVE MANAGEMENT

Interventions	Rationales
• Administer benzoyl peroxide, tretinoin, or a combination, as ordered.	• To control acne and reduce inflammation
• Administer a systemic antibiotic, as ordered.	• To treat persistent cases

OUTCOME:	EVALUATION CRITERIA:
• The child's acne outbreaks will be controlled.	• Lesions are reduced and free from infection.
	• The child complies with the health care regimen.

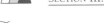

Patient Teaching

Educate the adolescent regarding the disease process, including the use of medical therapy.

Advise against the use of creams, oils, or cosmetics that may cause or aggravate acne.

Documentation

- Patient response to education and compliance with care regimen
- Extent of lesions
- Presence of pustules
- Signs of superinfection

Overview: Burns

Burn injuries are the third leading cause of accidental death in children. Most happen in the home and are preventable. Burns can be caused by thermal, chemical, electrical, or, rarely, radioactive agents.

Burns are classified as follows by depth:
- First degree—only the epidermis is involved; symptoms are pain and redness
- Second degree—epidermis and corium are involved; symptoms are pain, redness, and blisters
- Third degree—deep; full thickness; tough, light brown to black surface; dry; reduced sensitivity to touch or pain.

BURNS CLASSIFIED BY DEGREE

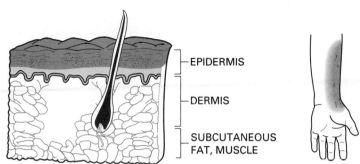

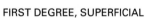

Skin Red, Dry

FIRST DEGREE, SUPERFICIAL

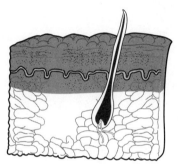

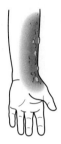

Blistered, Skin Moist, Pink or Red

SECOND DEGREE,
PARTIAL THICKNESS

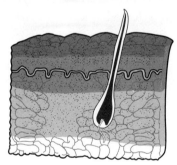

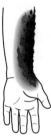

Charring, Skin Black, Brown, Red

THIRD DEGREE, FULL THICKNESS

NURSING DIAGNOSIS: IMPAIRED SKIN INTEGRITY

RELATED TO:
• *Burn trauma*

Nursing Interventions	Rationales
• Assess and support the airway and breathing process.	• To ensure adequate airway and ventilation
• Assess and support circulation.	• To ensure adequate circulating volume
• Assess for collateral injuries.	• To initiate appropriate interventions
• Shave hair from wound area, if needed.	• To facilitate healing
• Thoroughly clean the wound area.	• To reduce the risk of infection
• Be especially careful when handling the wound area.	• To preserve blisters intact, which reduces additional trauma to the skin
• Offer high-calorie, high-protein diet and snacks.	• To provide adequate nourishment for healing
• Prevent the child from scratching or picking at the wound.	• To keep the skin intact and reduce the risk of infection
• Position the child for minimal disturbance of the graft sites.	• To promote healing of skin grafts

COLLABORATIVE MANAGEMENT

Interventions	Rationales
• Begin I.V. fluid replacement.	• To prevent acute complications from fluid shifts and restore intravascular volume
• Debride burn area.	• To prevent infection, remove the dead tissue, and promote wound closure

NURSING DIAGNOSIS: IMPAIRED SKIN INTEGRITY (*CONTINUED*)

OUTCOME:
- The child's skin integrity will be restored.

EVALUATION CRITERIA:
- The wound heals properly.
- Skin grafts, if any, remain intact.
- The child experiences no additional complications.

NURSING DIAGNOSIS: PAIN

RELATED TO:
- *Discomfort caused by burn and treatment*

Nursing Interventions	Rationales
• Assess the child's pain medication requirements.	• To ensure adequate dosage to alleviate pain
• Assist the child to maintain a position of comfort.	• To ease pain and discomfort
• Instruct the child in the use of nonpharmacologic pain management techniques, if appropriate.	• To help control the child's reaction to pain
• Explain procedures honestly to the child and provide as much control as possible to the child during these procedures.	• To alleviate anxiety, increase the child's feeling of control, and ease pain
• Avoid touching or moving painful areas. Remove any irritants from the area.	• To reduce painful stimulation

COLLABORATIVE MANAGEMENT

Interventions	Rationales
• Administer pain medications, as ordered. Provide medications before the onset of pain or before any potentially uncomfortable procedures.	• To reduce pain and anxiety

NURSING DIAGNOSIS: PAIN (CONTINUED)

OUTCOME:
- The child's pain will be controlled adequately.

EVALUATION CRITERIA:
- The child reports the ability to tolerate the level of pain present.

- The child can rest comfortably.

NURSING DIAGNOSIS: HIGH RISK FOR INFECTION

RELATED TO:
- *Denuded skin and the presence of pathogenic organisms*

Nursing Interventions	Rationales
• Assess the child for fever.	• To identify the presence of infection
• Assess the wound for signs of infection, such as pus, erythematous borders, and foul-smelling drainage.	• To identify the presence of infection
• Implement and maintain strict infection control procedures.	• To reduce the risk of infection
• Avoid injury to the crust or eschar.	• To maintain the integrity of natural barriers to infection
• Isolate the child from other patients with upper respiratory tract or skin infections.	• To reduce the risk of infection
• Obtain wound culture results three times a week.	• To monitor for signs of increasing infection

COLLABORATIVE MANAGEMENT

Interventions	Rationales
• Apply topical antimicrobial ointments, as ordered.	• To resolve infection
• Administer systemic antibiotics, as ordered.	• To resolve infection

NURSING DIAGNOSIS: HIGH RISK FOR INFECTION *(CONTINUED)*

OUTCOME:	EVALUATION CRITERIA:
• The child will show no signs of wound infection.	• The burn site is free from signs of infection.
	• Wound culture results are normal.
	• The child's temperature and vital signs are normal.

Patient Teaching

Instruct the parents or caregivers regarding the management of burns, including signs of infection, and when to return for further medical treatment.

Instruct the parents or caregivers regarding dressing changes and the application of topical antimicrobial ointments.

Documentation

• Response to topical or systemic intervention
• Body surface area involvement of various burns
• Signs of infection (pus, drainage, erythema, fever)

Suggested Readings

Allison, M. "The Effects of Neurologic Injury on the Maturing Brain." *Headlines* (October/November 1992): 2–10.

Begley, Doreen K. "The Crying Infant." *Journal of Emergency Nursing* 20 (December 1994): 313.

Bobak, I. M., and M. D. Jensen. *Maternity and Gynecologic Care: The Nurse and the Family.* 5th ed. St. Louis: Mosby-Yearbook, 1993.

Brosnan, H. "Nursing Management of the Adolescent with Idiopathic Scoliosis." *Nursing Clinics of North America* 26 (March 1991): 17–31.

Burgess, A. W., and C. R. Hartman. "Children's Drawings." *Child Abuse and Neglect* 17 (January 1993): 161–168.

Burke, J. F. "From Desperation to Skin Regeneration: Progress in Burn Treatment." *Journal of Trauma* 30 (January 1990): 36–40.

Clark, E. B. "Congenital Heart Disease." In *Primary Pediatric Care,* edited by R. A. Hockuman et al. St. Louis: Mosby Yearbook, 1992.

Corey, M. Antoinette, and Ellen Rudy Clove. "Management of the Infant with RSV." *Journal of Pediatric Nursing* 6 (April 1991): 2.

Cusson, R. M. "Rice Based Oral Rehydration Fluid in the Treatment of Infant Diarrhea." *Journal of Pediatric Nursing* 7 (December 1992): 414–415.

Hahn, M. "Antibiotics for Children—An Overview." *Advance for Nurse Practitioners* 3 (February 1995): 25–28.

Kelley, S. J. *Pediatric Emergency Nursing.* 2nd ed. E. Norwalk, CT: Appleton & Lange, 1994.

Knipper, J. G. "Acute Poststreptococcal Glomerulonephritis." In *Pediatric Emergency Medicine,* edited by R. M. Barkin. St. Louis: Mosby, 1994.

Martinez, S. "Ambulatory Management of Burns in Children." *Journal of Pediatric Health Care* 6 (January 1992): 32–37.

Milinari, F. "Update on the Treatment of Pediculosis and Scabies." *Pediatric Nursing* 18 (November/December 1992): 600.

St. Pierre, Ann-Marie. "Triage Decisions: A Respiratory Emergency." *Journal of Emergency Nursing* 20 (August 1994): 338.

Suddaby, E., and S. Riker. "Defibrillation and Cardioversion in Children." *Pediatric Nursing* 17 (September/October 1991): 477–481.

Thomas, S. A., N. S. Rosenfield, J. M. Levanthal, and R. I. Markowitz. "Long Bone Fractures in Young Children: Distinguishing Accidental Injuries from Child Abuse." *Pediatrics* 88 (Supplement 1991): 471–476.

SECTION IV. COMMON PROBLEMS

ℰhapter 14. Fever

▽   ▽   ▽   ▽   ▽   ▽   ▽

Introduction

SEE TEXT PAGES

Fever is one of the most common chief complaints of parents who bring a child to a hospital emergency department or a pediatrician's office. Most children who need medical attention because of fever are less than 3 years of age. Common to this age-group are both minor and life-threatening infectious diseases, such as respiratory tract infection, occult bacteremia, and meningitis.

By itself, fever is not an illness, but it is a sign that accompanies various illnesses. Frequently, it is a common symptom of a nonemergent illness; however, it may be the only overt clue to a serious illness. To be considered fever, the body temperature must exceed what is considered the usual range of normal; with 98.6°F (37°C) deemed normal, a child with an oral temperature of 100.2°F (37.9°C) or a rectal reading exceeding 101°F (38°C) would be considered febrile.

The management of pediatric fever is controversial. Many nursing texts recommend aggressive fever management; others cite research evidence that fever is a normal physiologic process that has beneficial effects and does not necessarily require treatment. Antipyretics are the first line of treatment for fever, although they merely reduce the temperature and may have no effect on what is elevating it. Many believe that more clinical trials of commonly used fever treatments are needed.

Although often there is concern about brain damage, it is not caused solely by fever unless the temperature rises above 107°F (41.7°C).

POSSIBLE CAUSES OF FEVER IN CHILDREN

CAUSE	EXAMPLES
Bacterial Infection	• Bacteremia • Cellulitis • Meningitis • Osteomyelitis • Otitis media • Pneumonia • Pyelonephritis • Shigellosis • Urinary tract infection
Viral Illness	• Aseptic meningitis • Croup • Cytomegalovirus • Gastroenteritis • Upper respiratory tract infection
Collagen Vascular Disease	• Henoch-Schönlein purpura • Juvenile rheumatoid arthritis • Lupus erythematosus • Rheumatic fever
Drug Intoxication	• Amphetamines • Atropine • Phenothiazines • Phencyclidine hydrochloride • Salicylates
Cancers	• Hodgkin's lymphoma • Leukemia • Neuroblastoma • Sarcoma

Fever in a child includes the following physiologic and behavioral effects:
- Increased basal metabolism, which increases heart rate, respiratory rate, and oxygen demand
- Increased fluid and caloric requirements; each degree centigrade of fever raises caloric requirements by 12%
- Increased likelihood of dehydration caused by escalated insensible water loss, increased fluid requirements, and decreased intake

- Lowered seizure threshold and increased likelihood of febrile seizure in some children
- Lethargy and increased irritability

The febrile child with a history of seizures needs a special, detailed assessment. Although seizures in a child with fever are fairly common and usually represent an acute febrile illness that is not serious, they can indicate a serious CNS infection. The child who responds slowly or is postictal on arrival requires emergent management. Febrile children with a history of sickle cell disease or bronchopulmonary dysplasia and those who are immunocompromised or on immunosuppressive drug therapy have a higher incidence of serious illness.

NURSING DIAGNOSIS: HYPERTHERMIA

RELATED TO:
- *Increased metabolic rate, illness, or discomfort associated with febrile state*

Nursing Interventions	Rationales
• Assess temperature and other vital signs every 4 hours and as necessary.	• To monitor temperature and the child's response to interventions
• Administer an antipyretic (acetaminophen), as ordered. Monitor effectiveness for 30 to 60 minutes after it is given.	• To control fever
• After administering an antipyretic, give tepid sponge baths as prescribed for temperatures at or above 104°F (40°C) or those unresponsive to antipyretics.	• To reduce the child's elevated temperature through loss of body heat due to evaporation
• Dress the child in lightweight clothing and cover him or her lightly when in bed.	• To increase the child's comfort

NURSING DIAGNOSIS: HYPERTHERMIA (CONTINUED)

COLLABORATIVE MANAGEMENT

Interventions	Rationales
• Administer medications, as ordered: antibiotics, antipyretics.	• To control fever and reduce infection

NURSE ALERT:
A child younger than 3 months of age with a body temperature higher than 101°F (38.5°C) has a greater than 20-fold risk of serious infection when compared with an older child. Infants with high temperatures generally should be hospitalized and given antibiotics.

• After evaluation, including cultures of blood, urine, and cerebrospinal fluid, administer parenteral antibiotic therapy to hospitalized infants and children, as ordered.	• To ensure prompt treatment of children who are lethargic and showing signs of poor perfusion
• Instruct the caregivers of older children with temperatures less than 102.2°F (39°C) who do not appear toxic to return for additional evaluation if the fever persists for more than 2 days or if the child's condition deteriorates.	• To promote follow-up evaluation

NURSE ALERT:
Most studies indicate that bacteremia is most prevalent in children with higher temperatures (higher than 102.2°F [39°C]).

NURSING DIAGNOSIS: HYPERTHERMIA (CONTINUED)

OUTCOME:
- The child's temperature will return within the normal range and he or she will begin to resume normal behavior.

EVALUATION CRITERIA:
- The child maintains a normal temperature.
- The child reports feeling comfortable and begins to resume normal activity.
- The child gets adequate sleep and rest.

NURSING DIAGNOSIS: FLUID VOLUME DEFICIT

RELATED TO:
- *Dehydration caused by fluid loss through increased diaphoresis, evaporation, respiration, and body excretions resulting from the increased metabolism that accompanies the increase in the child's body temperature*

Nursing Interventions	Rationales
Monitor for signs of dehydration every 4 hours: - lack of tears - dry mucous membranes - poor skin turgor - sunken eyes - sunken fontanelle - increased pulse rate - decreased urination.	To anticipate the need for interventions
Maintain accurate intake and output records.	To determine actual fluid loss
Encourage fluid intake by using ice chips, ice pops, and flavored gelatin to replace fluids.	To promote adequate hydration
Weigh the child daily, being sure to use the same scale, at the same time of day, while the patient is wearing similar dress.	To monitor progress
Determine the amount of fluid required by the child.	To provide appropriate amounts of fluid

NURSING DIAGNOSIS: FLUID VOLUME DEFICIT (CONTINUED)

Nursing Interventions (Continued)	Rationales (Continued)
• Carefully monitor I.V. replacement therapy.	• To anticipate the need for increased fluid intake
• Provide favorite fluids, if possible.	• To promote fluid intake
• Encourage fluid consumption through game playing, the use of comic straws or cups, or other strategies.	• To increase the child's willingness to consume appropriate amounts of fluid
• Avoid tepid baths if there are signs of dehydration.	• To prevent an increase in vasoconstriction and heat retention, which raises the child's temperature and exacerbates dehydration

COLLABORATIVE MANAGEMENT

Interventions	Rationales
• Administer I.V. fluids, as necessary.	• To maintain normal fluid intake
• Administer antipyretic therapy.	• To reduce fever and accompanying irritability, which facilitates increased fluid intake

OUTCOME:	EVALUATION CRITERIA:
• The child's hydration levels will return to normal.	• The child has good skin turgor, moist membranes, flat fontanelles, adequate tear production, and normal pulse rate.
	• The child's intake and output are balanced.

NURSING DIAGNOSIS: KNOWLEDGE DEFICIT

RELATED TO:
• *Cause of the fever, care of the febrile child, and preventive and palliative measures*

Nursing Interventions	Rationales
• Instruct the parents or caregivers about factors related to fever in children. Include instruction about normal temperature ranges.	• To increase caregiver knowledge
• Teach the caregiver how to take an accurate temperature: - methods - timing - reading.	• To reassure caregivers that they are performing the procedure correctly and not hurting the child
• Explain that body temperature conforms to a normal diurnal cycle, with the lowest reading in the morning and the highest reading in the evening.	• To promote understanding of normal temperature variations
• Instruct caregivers about the use of aspirin. Explain contraindications for children under 16 years of age for varicella, flu (or flu-like symptoms), and viral illness.	• To provide information about the relation between aspirin and Reye's syndrome

COLLABORATIVE MANAGEMENT

Interventions	Rationales
• Describe the correct dose, method, and schedule as prescribed by the health care provider for administering antipyretics.	• To promote the correct use of medication to alleviate the symptoms of fever, even though the medication will not resolve the underlying cause

NURSING DIAGNOSIS: KNOWLEDGE DEFICIT (*CONTINUED*)

OUTCOME:

• The patient's caregivers will demonstrate a clearer understanding of the causes and care regimen for fever.

EVALUATION CRITERIA:

• The caregivers demonstrate an adequate understanding of:
  - what causes fever
  - misconceptions about fever
  - warning signs that should be reported to the health care provider.

• The caregivers demonstrate an understanding of the relation between Reye's syndrome and aspirin.

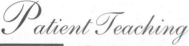

Reassure parents and other caregivers with "fever phobia" that fever is a common symptom of illness and that the way the child looks and acts is more important in identifying the degree of illness than is the degree of fever.

Fever is not something to be feared; it is a symptom of an illness that is often easily treated.

Discuss diagnostic tests with caregivers and the child, when appropriate. Explain the purpose of each test and why it is important in the assessment of the child.

Explain and reassure the caregiver and the child about any spinal taps to be done. Emphasize that the insertion site is below the level of the spinal cord and that there is little risk of paralysis.

Make sure the caregivers know if and how to call back for culture results.

Discuss any indicated antibiotic therapy.

Reinforce information about the avoidance of aspirin and its relevance to Reye's syndrome.

Provide specific follow-up instructions, including any conditions that necessitate re-evaluation.

Documentation

- General assessment, including level of consciousness and activity, color, skin turgor, rashes, and associated signs and symptoms
- Temperature on arrival, antipyretics given, and temperature on discharge or after antipyretics
- Treatment response
- Repeated pulse and respiratory rates when the child's temperature drops to ensure that these rates were elevated by fever and not by other causes
- Diagnostic tests done
- Teaching provided on follow-up care and fever control

Nursing Research

With the advent of tympanic membrane (TM) thermometry, many pediatric settings are using this quick and less invasive method for body temperature measurement. Results of a study of the accuracy of ear, rectal, and axillary readings as compared with core bladder temperatures showed a high correlation between bladder temperature and rectal temperature but a low correlation between axillary temperature and bladder temperature. TM temperatures correlated well but generally were lower by a mean of -0.3° to -0.7°C with deviation among children. Conclusions indicate that TM is a reasonable choice for routine temperature measurement in light of the speed, convenience, and acceptability of results.

Erickson, R. S., and T. M. Woo. "Accuracy of Infrared Ear Thermometry and Traditional Temperature Methods in Young Children." *Heart and Lung - The Journal of Critical Care* 23 (May/June 1994): 181–195.

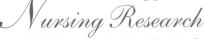

Chapter 15. Childhood Infections
▽ ▽ ▽ ▽ ▽ ▽ ▽

Introduction

SEE TEXT PAGES

Most childhood infections require interventions that focus on improving the child's comfort while the infection is resolved.

The following infections are discussed in this chapter:
• Chickenpox (varicella)
• Hepatitis
• Measles (rubeola)
• Mumps
• Rubella
• Scarlet fever and strep throat
• Epstein-Barr virus infection
• Whooping cough (pertussis)

When discussing common infectious diseases with the child's parents or other caregivers, stress these important points:
• Recommend appropriate immunization schedules.
• Explain immunization reactions and which require medical attention.
• Advise yearly immunization against influenza for chronically ill children.
• Instruct the parents or caregivers about methods they can use with their child to reduce pain and discomfort.
• Describe various diversional activities for an infected child.

Overview: Chickenpox

One of the most common childhood illnesses, chickenpox is a highly contagious viral infection that causes an itchy, vesicular rash that may cover most of the body. The rash is diffusely spread, and the lesions are often in various stages of healing.

After a 10- to 20-day incubation period, there is a period of mild variable fever and malaise for about 24 hours before the rash appears. The course of the disease is usually uncomplicated, and treatment focuses on symptomatic relief of pruritus and infection prevention.

NURSING DIAGNOSIS: KNOWLEDGE DEFICIT

RELATED TO:

• *Treatment and management of varicella infection*

Nursing Interventions	Rationales
• Review the goals of therapy with the child's parents or caregivers: - Prevent exposure to infectious agents. - Promote the child's comfort. - Encourage frequent bathing, especially oatmeal baths.	• To provide methods for promoting the child's comfort
• Dress the child in loose, comfortable clothing.	• To keep the skin clean, limit the child's access for scratching, and promote comfort
• Trim the child's fingernails.	• To reduce the risk of injury if the child does scratch his or her pox

COLLABORATIVE MANAGEMENT

Interventions	Rationales
• Administer antipyretics, as ordered.	• To reduce fever
• Administer an antihistamine, as ordered.	• To control pruritus
• Treat the affected areas topically with calamine lotion, as ordered.	• To relieve itching
• Administer antibiotics, as ordered.	• To treat bacterial skin lesion superinfection

OUTCOME:

• The child will be free from infection and able to rest comfortably.

EVALUATION CRITERIA:

• Pruritus is controlled.

• Skin lesions heal without infection.

Patient Teaching

Caution parents or caregivers to restrict the child's contact with noninfected people.

Advise the parents or caregivers to keep the child from school or day care until all lesions have dried (about 7 days).

Discourage the use of aspirin for easing discomfort because its use has been linked to Reye's syndrome.

Documentation

- Character and distribution of lesions
- Isolation status while the child is in the health care facility
- Signs of infection around skin lesions

Overview: Hepatitis

Hepatitis is an inflammation of the liver that is caused by a virus. The disease is treated symptomatically and is usually self-limiting, unless chronic hepatitis develops.

Both hepatitis A and hepatitis B are communicable from a few days to 1 month or more after onset of symptoms.

Manifestations of the disease occur rapidly and vary considerably.

The symptoms for type B are like those for hepatitis A infections, but unlike hepatitis A, they manifest more slowly.

NURSING DIAGNOSIS: ALTERED NUTRITION (LESS THAN BODY REQUIREMENTS)

RELATED TO:
- *Anorexia, nausea, and vomiting*

Nursing Interventions	Rationales
• Assess the child's normal eating patterns, including likes and dislikes.	• To provide baseline information
• Provide small, frequent meals. Offer the child's favorite foods.	• To promote eating

Nursing Interventions *(Continued)*

- Allow the child to make his or her own dietary choices.

- Monitor I.V. fluids.

- Maintain strict intake and output measurements.

Rationales *(Continued)*

- To increase patient involvement in the care regimen

- To provide short-term replacement for fluid loss from diarrhea

- To monitor hydration status

COLLABORATIVE MANAGEMENT

Interventions

- Consult with the dietitian, if required, to provide a high-calorie, high-protein, high-carbohydrate, low-fat diet.

- Administer parenteral fluids, as ordered.

Rationales

- To ensure adequate nutrition

- To maintain hydration

OUTCOME:

- The child will maintain adequate levels of nutrition for growth and development.

EVALUATION CRITERIA:

- The child's weight is adequate for his or her age and frame size.

- Hydration status is adequate.

Patient Teaching

Advise the parents or caregivers about good sanitation and personal hygiene practices, particularly careful hand washing after changing diapers, helping the older child with toileting, or sanitary disposal of feces.

Recommend that environmental sanitary precautions be taken because the virus may remain on objects for some time.

Dishes and linens should be cleaned in hot soapy water.

Recommend immunization against hepatitis B in infants.

Inform the parents or caregivers to use medications only under the advice of the health care provider because many drugs are metabolized by the liver.

Documentation

- Intake and output
- Daily weight
- Color of urine and stool
- Enteric precautions taken

Overview: Measles (Rubeola)

Measles is an acute disease transmitted by direct contact with infectious droplets or by airborne spread.

NURSING DIAGNOSIS: PAIN

RELATED TO:
- *Infection, fever, parotitis, and photophobia*

Nursing Interventions	Rationales
• Maintain bed rest and decrease activity level.	• To promote adequate rests
• Keep lights dimmed.	• To reduce photophobia
• Provide the child with frequent tepid baths and saline irrigation of the eyes.	• To reduce discomfort from itching
• Dress the child in loose cotton clothing.	• To avoid skin irritation

COLLABORATIVE MANAGEMENT

Interventions	Rationales
• Administer antipyretics, as ordered.	• To control fever
• Administer immune globulin after exposure.	• To prevent additional complications
• Administer antibiotics, as ordered.	• To resolve infection

NURSING DIAGNOSIS: PAIN (CONTINUED)

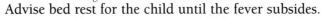

OUTCOME:
- The child will get adequate rest and experience minimal pain and discomfort.

EVALUATION CRITERIA:
- Signs of infection are absent.

- The child expresses that pain and discomfort are lessened.

Patient Teaching

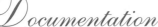

Advise bed rest for the child until the fever subsides.

Instruct the parents or caregivers to keep the child from school or day care for 7 days after the onset of the rash.

Exposed children should be immunized prophylactically with immune globulin.

Documentation

- Presentation and character of rash
- Response to interventions
- Report measles case to the local health department

Overview: Mumps

Mumps, caused by the paramyxovirus, occurs worldwide and spreads by direct contact or aerosolization of respiratory secretions and through fomites. Humans are its only known natural host.

Mumps primarily affects the salivary glands. The parotid, sublingual, and submaxillary glands may be involved. Orchitis and oophoritis may occur in the older child.

The illness is self-limiting unless complications ensue. Complications are infrequent in children or adolescents.

NURSING DIAGNOSIS: PAIN

RELATED TO:
• *Parotitis*

Nursing Interventions	Rationales
• Apply heat or cold to salivary glands.	• To reduce discomfort
• Provide a liquid diet or soft foods.	• To eliminate or reduce the need for chewing food
• Avoid acidic foods.	• To prevent irritation

COLLABORATIVE MANAGEMENT

Interventions	Rationales
• Administer antipyretics, as ordered.	• To reduce fever
• Administer analgesics, as ordered.	• To reduce pain

OUTCOME:	EVALUATION CRITERIA:
• The child will experience reduced or no pain.	• The child reports a reduction or absence of pain.
	• The child gets adequate rest and can rest in comfort.

Patient Teaching

Advise bed rest for the child until swelling subsides.

Teach parents or caregivers comfort measures to use at home.

NURSE ALERT:
Complications such as orchitis, pancreatitis, nephritis, myocarditis, and meningoencephalitis require further medical and nursing management.

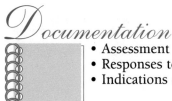

Documentation
- Assessment findings
- Responses to interventions
- Indications of complications

Overview: Rubella

Rubella is usually a mild disease, chiefly transmitted through direct or droplet contact from nasopharyngeal secretions. It is relatively uncommon today because of effective vaccination. It is important to protect pregnant women from infection to prevent congenital rubella, which causes a number of birth defects and chronic infection. Mental retardation, cardiac anomalies, and various other birth defects are seen.

Care providers should ensure that testing and vaccination services are available to protect from intrauterine and congenital rubella and prevent spontaneous abortion, stillbirth, and congenital rubella syndrome.

NURSING DIAGNOSIS: KNOWLEDGE DEFICIT

RELATED TO:
- *Disease process and goals of treatment*

Nursing Interventions	Rationales
• Provide parents or caregivers information about: - symptoms - duration of illness - communicability.	• To increase understanding
• Stress the importance of isolating the infected child from any pregnant women.	• To reduce the risk of infection for the mother and fetus

COLLABORATIVE MANAGEMENT

Interventions	Rationales
• Administer antipyretics, as ordered.	• To reduce fever
• Administer antihistamines, as ordered.	• To control itching

NURSING DIAGNOSIS: KNOWLEDGE DEFICIT (*CONTINUED*)

OUTCOME:
- The child's infection will be resolved.

EVALUATION CRITERIA:
- Vital signs are normal.
- The child expresses a return to levels of comfort.

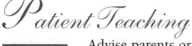

Advise parents or caregivers that immunization of girls should be done before puberty. Immunization after puberty should only be done if pregnancy has been ruled out.

Caution the parents or caregivers to keep the child from school or day care for 7 days after onset of rash.

Women who are not vaccinated are advised not to become pregnant for 2 to 3 months after vaccination.

Documentation

- Maternal rubella immunity in pregnant females

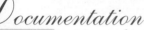

Overview: Scarlet Fever and Strep Throat

A child with strep throat may also develop the rash known as scarlet fever or scarlatina, caused by infection with group A streptococci. This characteristic rash appears 24 to 48 hours after the onset of pharyngitis. Rheumatic fever, whose incidence has significantly declined, is also due to streptococcal infection.

Strep throat. After a 2- to 4-day incubation period, the child develops tonsillitis, fever, headache, and malaise, after which the rash appears. The rash consists of red, pinpoint maculopapular lesions on the chest, extremities, and joint folds. The tongue has a thick white coating with inflamed papillae showing beneath it. After 4 to 5 days, the tongue peels, leaving a strawberry appearance; the rash fades in a few days.

Rheumatic fever. One to 3 weeks after a throat infection, the child develops a fever, malaise, and acute migratory polyarthritis. Carditis commonly develops.

NURSING DIAGNOSIS: PAIN

RELATED TO:
- *Infection*

Nursing Interventions	Rationales
• Encourage adequate fluid intake. Clear fluids and soft foods are easiest to tolerate.	• To provide adequate nutrition
• Provide warm throat irrigations or lozenges for the older child.	• To decrease discomfort
• Apply warm or cold compresses to the child's neck.	• To reduce swelling of the cervical nodes

COLLABORATIVE MANAGEMENT

Interventions	Rationales
• Administer antipyretics, as ordered.	• To reduce fever
• Administer penicillin or, for the penicillin-sensitive child, erythromycin, as ordered.	• To resolve bacterial infection

OUTCOME:
- The child will experience a reduction in pain.

EVALUATION CRITERIA:
- Vital signs are normal.
- The child expresses a return to levels of comfort.

Patient Teaching

Discuss the treatment regimen with the parents or caregivers.

Institute precautions to prevent the spread of disease for the first 24 hours of treatment.

Advise the parents or caregivers to seek medical evaluation if fever still persists 24 hours after antibiotics have been initiated.

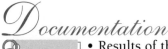

Documentation

• Results of throat culture

Overview: Epstein-Barr Virus Infection

The Epstein-Barr virus causes infectious mononucleosis, which commonly affects the oropharynx, causing lymphadenopathy.

NURSING DIAGNOSIS: PAIN

RELATED TO:
• *Fever, malaise, and sore throat*

Nursing Interventions	Rationales
• Instruct the parents or caregivers to avoid the use of aspirin for pain control.	• To reduce the risk of Reye's syndrome
• Assess for abdominal tenderness or shoulder pain.	• To identify early signs of complications
• Assist the child to maintain a comfortable position.	• To decrease discomfort
• Encourage the child to sleep by creating a calm, restful environment.	• To promote adequate rest, which speeds recovery
• Instruct the patient to complete range-of-motion exercises.	• To reduce muscle stiffness

COLLABORATIVE MANAGEMENT

Interventions	Rationales
• Administer antipyretics, as ordered.	• To reduce fever
• Administer analgesics, as ordered.	• To alleviate pain

NURSING DIAGNOSIS: PAIN (CONTINUED)

OUTCOME:
- The child will experience little or no pain.

EVALUATION CRITERIA:
- The child reports a reduction in pain.

- The child gets adequate rest and can rest comfortably.

- Indications of complications are absent.

Patient Teaching

Provide information regarding the cause and disease course.

Emphasize the need for adequate rest.

Alert the parents or caregivers to signs of complications, such as hepatitis and idiopathic thrombocytopenia.

Reinforce the need for health care provider follow-up to assess any complications.

Documentation

- Assessment findings
- Results of monospot test

Overview: Whooping Cough (Pertussis)

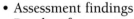

Whooping cough begins with mild upper respiratory tract symptoms and can progress to severe paroxysms of cough.

Clinical manifestations include coryza, dry cough that worsens at night. Cough is characterized by paroxysms of several sharp coughs in one expiration followed by a rapid deep inspiration and a "whoop." During these episodes, the child may be cyanotic and diaphoretic. The child may have dyspnea or fever, and vomiting may occur after a coughing spell.

NURSING DIAGNOSIS: INEFFECTIVE BREATHING PATTERN

RELATED TO:
- *Severe cough*

Nursing Interventions	Rationales
• Provide warm, humidified air or oxygen.	• To decrease drying of mucous membranes and relieve cough
• Reduce other cough stimuli, when possible.	• To decrease coughing spasms
• Promote adequate rest.	• To prevent coughing episodes and promote healing
• Isolate the child during the infectious period.	• To reduce the spread of infection

COLLABORATIVE MANAGEMENT

Interventions	Rationales
• Administer erythromycin, as ordered.	• To resolve infection
• Administer oxygen and suction secretions, as needed.	• To ensure adequate oxygenation
• Provide tube feeding, as ordered.	• To ensure adequate nutrition

OUTCOME:	EVALUATION CRITERIA:
• The child will maintain adequate ventilation through an effective breathing pattern.	• The child's cough lessens.
	• The child receives adequate rest.

Patient Teaching

Advise the parents or caregivers that the effects of immunization are not lifelong.

Discuss the need for isolation during the infectious period.

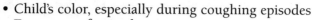

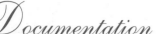 ocumentation

- Child's color, especially during coughing episodes
- Frequency of episodes
- General level of respiratory distress
- Isolation status

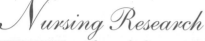 ursing Research

Through discussion groups composed of parents or caregivers whose children were ill with varicella, the researchers identified three types of disturbance in family function. They are as follows:
- Parental distress
- Behavioral changes in the sick child
- General disruption of family arrangements

Conclusions support the idea that disruption is considerable during the first days of an illness and declines over a 2-week period. These findings indicate that nursing interventions need to address the family's need for guidance in coping with disruptions.

McKenna, S. P., and S. M. Hunt. "A Measure of Family Disruption for Use in Chicken Pox and Other Childhood Illnesses." *Social Science and Medicine* 38, no. 5 (1994): 725–731.

Chapter 16. Poisoning and Ingestions

▽ ▽ ▽ ▽ ▽ ▽ ▽

Introduction

SEE TEXT PAGES

Accidental poisoning is a major health care problem in the United States that frequently brings the child to the emergency department for treatment. Most children will not be permanently harmed if immediate treatment is given. More than 63% of poisonings occur in children younger than 5 years of age. Poisoning can involve an ingested, inhaled, or absorbed material.

DRUG INTOXICATION SIGNS AND SYMPTOMS

SIGNS AND SYMPTOMS	TOXIN
Hyperthermia	• Aspirin • Acetaminophen • Amphetamines • Anticholinergics • Atropine • Beta blockers • Organophosphates • Alcohol or narcotic withdrawal
Hypothermia	• Alcohol • Anesthetics • Barbiturates • Carbon monoxide • Narcotics • Phenothiazines • Tricyclic antidepressants
Tachycardia	• Amphetamines • Phencyclidine (PCP) • Sympathomimetics • Thyroid replacement drugs • Narcotic withdrawal

DRUG INTOXICATION SIGNS AND SYMPTOMS (CONTINUED)

SIGNS AND SYMPTOMS	TOXIN
Bradycardia	• Beta blockers • Calcium channel blockers • Clonidine • Digitalis
Depressed respirations	• Alcohol • Sedatives • Hypnotics • Narcotics
Increased respirations	• Amphetamines • Ethylene glycol or methanol salicylates • Hydrocarbon pulmonary aspiration • Phenothiazines • Theophylline
Hypertension	• Amphetamines • Nicotine • PCP • Sympathomimetics • Tricyclic antidepressants • Narcotic or sedative withdrawal
Hypotension	• Beta blockers • Sedatives • Hypnotics • Narcotics • Tricyclic antidepressants
Seizures	• Aminophylline • Caffeine • Cocaine • Lidocaine • Narcotics • Sedatives • Pesticides • Tricyclic antidepressants

DRUG INTOXICATION SIGNS AND SYMPTOMS (CONTINUED)

SIGNS AND SYMPTOMS	TOXIN
Psychotic reactions	• Hallucinogens (PCP/LSD) • Heavy metals • Sympathomimetics
Small pupils (miosis)	• Barbiturates • Cholinergics • Clonidine • Narcotics
Large pupils (mydriasis)	• Anticholinergics
Salivation, lacrimation, urination, defecation, GI cramps, and emesis	• Cholinergics
Sweating, salivation, miosis, muscle fasciculation, and bradycardia	• Organophosphates • Carbamates

NURSING DIAGONOSIS: HIGH RISK FOR INJURY

RELATED TO:
• *Ingestion or exposure to toxic substance*

Nursing Interventions	Rationales
• Support the child's ABCs: airway, breathing, and circulation.	• To stabilize the child's condition
• Identify the poison ingested, if possible.	• To guide the treatment plan

NURSE ALERT:
Emesis is contraindicated with the ingestion of corrosive agents (such as acids or alkali) because it may result in oral, esophageal, and gastric erosion.

Nursing Interventions *(Continued)*

- Provide symptomatic care for associated conditions, such as warming to address hypothermia.

Rationales *(Continued)*

- To treat secondary conditions

COLLABORATIVE MANAGEMENT

Interventions

- Administer oxygen, as ordered.

- Assist in intubation and mechanical ventilation procedures.

- Secure and maintain I.V. access.

- Install cardiac and/or oxygen monitors.

- Perform gastric lavage, as ordered.

- Administer activated charcoal, as ordered.

- Administer ipecac syrup, as ordered.

Rationales

- To maximize gas exchange

- To ensure patent airway and adequate ventilation

- To provide route for administration of I.V. fluid or medication, as required

- To monitor vital functions

- To prevent or decrease poison absorption by removing poison from the child's stomach

- To bind with some poisons

- To induce vomiting

NURSE ALERT:
Administration of ipecac is contraindicated in a child with or at risk for a rapidly deteriorating level of consciousness because he or she cannot protect the airway.

- Provide whole bowel irrigation with cathartic, as ordered.

- Secure and maintain orogastric or nasogastric tube, as ordered.

- To expedite poison elimination

- To reduce aspiration risk and perform lavage

NURSING DIAGONOSIS: HIGH RISK FOR INJURY (CONTINUED)

COLLABORATIVE MANAGEMENT (CONTINUED)

Interventions (Continued)

- Administer naloxone, as ordered.

- Consult with health care providers who specialize in toxicology, as needed,

- Initiate hemodialysis or hemoperfusion, as ordered.

Rationales (Continued)

- To treat respiratory depression, which may be the result of narcotic ingestion

- To acquire additional information

- To expedite poison elimination

OUTCOME:

- The child will maintain adequate vital functions and will recover from the effects of poison ingestion.

EVALUATION CRITERIA:

- The toxin is cleared from the child's body.

- The child maintains adequate ventilation.

- Blood pressure and pulse rate are normal.

- Vital signs are normal.

Patient Teaching

Instruct the parents or caregivers about poisoning prevention:
- Lock all medications in a cabinet out of the child's reach.
- Use child-resistant containers for all prescription or over-the-counter drugs.
- Never call medications given to a child "candy."
- Dispose of household cleaning products properly.
- Keep all items in their original containers, locking them in a secure cabinet after each use.
- Never mix household bleach with a toilet bowel cleaner or ammonia.
- Emphasize that nonprescription drugs, such as vitamins, aspirin, and acetaminophen, are just as dangerous as prescription drugs.
- Identify other sources of poison, such as cosmetics, perfumes, and plants.

Provide the telephone number of the local poison control center, and remind the parents or caregivers to keep it readily available. Stress that it should be used whenever poisoning is suspected.

Inform the parents or caregivers about the danger of the child taking medications that they may be taking, such as the following:
• Tricyclic antidepressants, such as Elavil, Norpramin, and Tofranil
• 4-Aminoquinolines, such as Aralen and Plaquenil
• Antidiarrheals, such as Lomotil and Motofen
• Hydrocodone-based cough syrups, such as Tussionex
• Propoxyphene, such as Darvon and Darvocet
• Ethchlorvynol, such as Placidyl
• Lindane, such as Kwell
• Lithium carbonate, such as Eskalith and Lithobid
• Glyburide and glipizide, such as DiaBeta and Micronase-Glucotrol
• Clonidine, such as Catapres

Remind the parents or caregivers that these medications are formulated for adult use and that severe adverse reactions can occur if administered to children.

Documentation

• Substance ingested, time, amount, and interventions
• Serial assessment, use of cardiorespiratory monitors
• Drug levels

$\mathcal{C}$hapter 17. Trauma

▽　▽　▽　▽　▽　▽　▽

$\mathcal{I}$ntroduction

SEE TEXT PAGES

Injuries are the leading cause of death in children; each year about 25,000 children in the United States die of injuries. An estimated 600,000 children are hospitalized owing to injury, and about 16 million children are treated for injuries in a hospital emergency department.

Motor vehicle–related trauma is the most common cause of injuries. It is responsible for 63% of all pediatric deaths, and together with falls, it is responsible for 80% to 90% of blunt trauma to children.

The child's skull is malleable and offers limited protection to brain tissue. It is relatively large and heavy compared with body size, increasing the likelihood of head trauma from acceleration-deceleration forces.

Drowning and near-drowning are the leading causes of death in the infant-to-3-year-old age-group. Other causes of pediatric trauma include fires and burns, firearms, and poisoning.

The type and degree of trauma to a child depend on a number of elements, including the mechanism of injury; developmental factors, such as age, anatomy, and physiology; and psychosocial factors.

MANAGING CHILDHOOD TRAUMATIC INJURY

AGE AND DEVELOPMENTAL CONCERN	COMMON INJURY	INTERVENTIONS
Birth to 12 months	• Falls	• Involve the parents or caregivers in the infant's care.
• Increased mobility	• Foreign-body aspiration	• Obtain a complete history.

MANAGING CHILDHOOD TRAUMATIC INJURY (CONTINUED)

AGE AND DEVELOPMENTAL CONCERN	COMMON INJURY	INTERVENTIONS
12 months to 3 years • Need for environmental exploration • No concept of danger	• Poisonings • Falls • Playground injuries • Burns • Near-drowning • Foreign-body aspiration	• Do not separate the child from the parents or caregiver. • Allow the caregiver to hold and comfort the child. • Use a quiet and reassuring tone and simple words and phrases.
3 to 5 years • More group activities	• Less parental supervision • Falls • Playground injuries • Ingestion	• Keep the child and parents or caregivers together. • Explain procedures clearly and concisely. • Cover external injuries with adhesive bandages or dressings. • Allow the child to handle equipment.
6 to 12 years • Increasing independence • Ties to peers develop	• Sports- and play-related injuries • Bicycle-related injuries	• Maintain privacy. • Allow the child to participate in care. • Explain all procedures. • Be honest. • Obtain a history from the patient when possible.

MANAGING CHILDHOOD TRAUMATIC INJURY (CONTINUED)

AGE AND DEVELOPMENTAL CONCERN	COMMON INJURY	INTERVENTIONS
Teenagers • Need for peer acceptance • Lack of judgment • Oriented to present • Risk-takers	• Motor vehicle–related injuries • Substance abuse • Suicide attempts	• Maintain privacy. • Explain all procedures. • Answer questions honestly. • Obtain a history from the patient. • Be aware of family dynamics.

NURSING DIAGNOSIS: HIGH RISK FOR INJURY

RELATED TO:
• *Trauma*

Nursing Interventions	Rationales
Airway and Cervical Spine Trauma • Open the airway, using jaw-thrust/chin-lift method.	• To prevent hyperextension of the cervical spine
• Suction the oropharynx.	• To remove vomitus, blood, or teeth, if present
• Insert an oral or nasal airway, if indicated.	• To maintain a patent airway
Breathing • Assess respiratory status.	• To identify signs of impending respiratory failure

• Auscultate for breath sounds in these locations:
  - over trachea
  - bilateral anterior aspect of chest
  - epigastrium
  - high in axillar region
	• To obtain an accurate respiratory evaluation and determine the extent of injuries

Nursing Interventions *(Continued)*	Rationales *(Continued)*
• Administer supplemental oxygen, as needed.	• To ensure adequate oxygenation
• Assist with ventilation efforts.	• To maintain adequate ventilation and gas exchange
• Insert a nasogastric or an orogastric tube, as needed.	• To prevent aspiration of stomach contents and decompress the abdomen

Circulation

• Assess apical pulse, including rate, rhythm, and quality.	• To identify signs of complications
• Assess capillary refill time.	• To identify signs of inadequate perfusion
• Place a pneumatic antishock garment on the child, if suitable.	• To shunt blood to vital organs

NURSE ALERT:
Exercise caution in using these devices. Do not inflate the abdominal compartment because this may inhibit respiratory excursion in children.

• Administer fluids, as ordered. Secure and maintain large-bore I.V. lines.	• To begin fluid resuscitation
• Administer blood products, as needed.	• To restore volume

Disability

• Assess neurologic function, including Glasgow Coma Scale rating.	• To determine the baseline and identify neurologic injuries
• Assist with intubation or hyperventilation in cases of severe head injury.	• To maintain arterial carbon dioxide pressure of 20 to 25 mm Hg

NURSING DIAGNOSIS: HIGH RISK FOR INJURY (CONTINUED)

Nursing Interventions (Continued)

Rationales (Continued)

Disability (continued)
- Maintain cervical spine stability.
  - To prevent injury to the cervical spine

- Apply a cervical collar.
  - To immobilize the child's neck and prevent additional injury

- Elevate the head of the bed once cervical spine injuries have been ruled out.
  - To decrease intracranial pressure

Thermoregulation
- Use radiant warmers, warm blankets, warm I.V. fluids, and warm blood products.
  - To prevent hypothermia

Gastrointestinal and Genitourinary Injuries
- Assess the abdomen for tenderness, distention, and indications of injury.
  - To determine the extent of injury

- Insert a nasogastric or an orogastric tube.
  - To prevent the aspiration of stomach contents, decompress the abdomen, and reduce the pressure of the stomach on the child's diaphragm

- Measure nasogastric output and assess for the presence of blood.
  - To record accurate output and identify indications of complications

- Insert an indwelling catheter, if needed, once genitourinary injury has been ruled out.
  - To monitor urine output

- Perform a urine dipstick test for the presence of blood.
  - To assess for urinary tract trauma

Musculoskeletal Injuries
- Assess the child's pelvis for instability.
  - To determine the extent of the injuries

Nursing Interventions *(Continued)*   Rationales *(Continued)*
Musculoskeletal Injuries *(continued)*

- Assess the child's legs for deformities and injuries.
  - To determine the extent of the injuries

- Monitor the neurovascular status of the injured extremities.
  - To identify signs of circulatory impairment or compartment syndrome

- Splint the injured extremities.
  - To promote comfort and reduce the risk of additional injury

- Assess the child's back for tenderness along the spine or flank tenderness.
  - To identify the extent of the injuries

- Assess the child's tetanus immunization status. Administer a booster shot, as needed.
  - To prevent tetanus infection

Psychosocial Factors

- Stand so that the child can see you clearly. Speak slowly and clearly in a comforting voice. Avoid using words that are indicative of death, dismemberment, or mutilation.
  - To reduce the child's anxiety and fears about:
    - losing control
    - mutilation
    - death
    - disfigurement
    - pain
    - getting into trouble with parents or caregivers

- Describe your care activities in age-appropriate terms. Be honest about painful procedures.
  - To promote a trust relationship between you and the child

- Avoid talking about the child or other family members as if the child were not there.
  - To alleviate the child's anxiety

- Use nonpharmacologic pain control methods until pain medications can be safely administered.
  - To control pain and discomfort

- Encourage the parents or caregivers to remain with the child and offer comfort.
  - To alleviate the child's fears and anxiety and to prepare the parents or caregivers for helping the child

NURSING DIAGNOSIS: HIGH RISK FOR INJURY (CONTINUED)

COLLABORATIVE MANAGEMENT

Interventions	Rationales
• Insert an endotracheal tube, if required.	• To ensure adequate respiration
• Assist with intubation or hyperventilation, as ordered.	• To maintain arterial carbon dioxide pressure of 20 to 25 mm Hg
• Administer atropine, as ordered.	• To prevent bradycardia during intubation
• Administer paralytics or sedatives, as ordered.	• To restrict the child's mobility and reduce the risk of accidental extubation
• Obtain a chest radiograph, as ordered.	• To assess chest injuries and ensure correct placement of the endotracheal tube
• Assist in the insertion of chest tubes, as ordered.	• To treat hemothorax, pneumothorax, or hemopneumothorax
• Administer lactated Ringer's solution, as ordered.	• To replace volume
• Administer osmotic diuretics, such as mannitol, as ordered.	• To reduce intracranial pressure
• Obtain cervical spine, chest, pelvic, or extremity radiographs, as ordered.	• To identify the extent of the child's injuries
• Administer prophylactic antibiotics, as ordered.	• To reduce the risk of infection

NURSE ALERT:
Be sure to explain the child's condition and the treatment procedures being used before the parents or caregivers see the child.

COLLABORATIVE MANAGEMENT (CONTINUED)

Interventions (Continued)

• Provide frequent updates about the child's condition. Refer the parents or caregivers to appropriate social workers for additional assistance.

Rationales (Continued)

• To address parental or caregiver concerns

OUTCOME:

• The child's injuries will be accurately assessed and appropriate treatments will be initiated.

EVALUATION CRITERIA:

• The child's pain is under control as evidenced by the child's report and the absence of objective signs of pain, such as crying, splinting the injured area, and facial grimacing.

• Vital signs are stable.

• Signs of shock are reduced or absent.

Patient Teaching

Avoid discussing preventive measures with the parents or caregivers of a child who is severely injured.

When appropriate, discuss accident prevention, including the following:
• Always use child safety seats while driving.
• Instruct children in safety habits to follow when bike riding.
• Teach water safety. Emphasize the importance of remaining with children who are swimming or playing in water.
• Stress the importance of firearm safety.

Documentation

• Primary and secondary assessment findings
• Serial vital signs
• Ongoing assessment
• Response to interventions
• Glasgow Coma Scale ratings
• Pediatric trauma scores

Chapter 18. Shock

▽ ▽ ▽ ▽ ▽ ▽ ▽

Introduction

SEE TEXT PAGES

Shock is a circulatory disturbance with systemic imbalance between oxygen supply and demand. Without prompt treatment, this imbalance results in impaired cellular, tissue, and organ function with subsequent death. The major categories of pediatric shock are hypovolemic, distributive, and cardiogenic.

NURSING DIAGNOSIS: ALTERED TISSUE PERFUSION

RELATED TO:
• *Hypovolemia*

Nursing Interventions	Rationales
• Monitor the child's cardiorespiratory status.	• To identify signs of respiratory insufficiency or cardiac arrhythmias
• Administer high-flow oxygen.	• To promote oxygenation
• Secure and maintain I.V. access.	• To provide an administration route for medications and fluid
• Maintain intake and output records.	• To identify signs of inadequate hydration and to track fluid resuscitation and response
• Insert a urinary catheter. Monitor urine output.	• To assess renal tissue perfusion and urinary function
• Monitor neurologic status.	• To identify signs of inadequate cerebral tissue perfusion
• Determine the source of volume loss and control the bleeding.	• To prevent further losses
• Assist with arterial line insertion, as indicated.	• To monitor systemic pressure

COLLABORATIVE MANAGEMENT

Interventions	Rationales
• Administer I.V. fluids, as ordered.	• To replace volume
• Administer vasopressors, as ordered, once volume is restored. Rapid I.V. fluid bolus of Ringer's lactate or 0.9% normal saline solution (20 mL/kg) may be appropriate.	• To increase blood pressure and improve perfusion
• Administer blood products, as ordered.	• To replace volume and increase oxygen-carrying capacity

OUTCOME:	EVALUATION CRITERIA:
• The child will maintain adequate tissue perfusion.	• The child's level of consciousness is normal or shows signs of improving.
	• Vital signs are normal or improving.
	• Skin color and warmth are normal.
	• Capillary refill time is within normal ranges.

NURSING DIAGNOSIS: HIGH RISK FOR INFECTION

RELATED TO:
• *Septic shock*

Nursing Interventions	Rationales
• Assess possible sources of infection, such as: - lungs - genitourinary system - GI system - I.V. catheters.	• To identify the source of sepsis

NURSING DIAGNOSIS: HIGH RISK FOR INFECTION (CONTINUED)

Nursing Interventions *(Continued)*

- Monitor the child's temperature and take measures to maintain it in the normal range, such as:
  - using a cooling mattress
  - administering tepid sponge baths
  - limiting the number of blankets on the child.

- Obtain laboratory culture and sensitivity results.

- Monitor the child for signs of drug toxicity.

- Initiate isolation measures.

Rationales *(Continued)*

- To identify signs of increasing infection and reduce cardiovascular stress

- To determine the effectiveness of interventions and to identify worsening infection

- To prevent toxic effects

- To reduce the risk of infection

COLLABORATIVE MANAGEMENT

Interventions

- Administer antibiotics, as ordered.

- Remove possible sources of infection, as ordered, such as I.V. lines.

- Assist with wound drainage procedures.

Rationales

- To resolve the infection

- To eliminate the source of sepsis

- To eliminate the source of sepsis

OUTCOME:

- The child's infection will be resolved.

EVALUATION CRITERIA:

- The cause of infection is identified and eliminated.

- Vital signs are normal.

- The child's wound, if there is one, shows signs of healing.

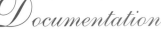

Patient Teaching

Explain all equipment and procedures. Answer all questions thoroughly.

Prepare the parents or caregivers and the child for hospital admission.

Documentation

- Vital signs
- Cardiovascular assessment
- Neurologic assessment
- Response to fluid boluses and vasopressors
- Intake and output

Suggested Readings

Bocchino, C. "Immunizing America's Children." *Pediatric Nursing* 19 (May/June 1993): 281–282.

Cherry, J. D., and R. D. Fleigin, eds. *Textbook of Pediatric Infectious Disease.* 3rd ed. Philadelphia: W. B. Saunders, 1992.

Deason, J. G. "Case Review: Acute Iron Ingestion in a 2-Year-Old Child." *Journal of Emergency Nursing* 21 (February 1995): 9–11.

Farrington, E. "Acyclovir in the Treatment of Chickenpox." *Pediatric Nursing* 18 (September/October 1992): 499–503.

Grimes, D. E., and L. F. Woolbert. "Facts and Fallacies About Streptococcal Infection and Rheumatic Fever." *Journal of Pediatric Health Care* 4 (July/August 1990): 186–192.

Gurevich, I., R. A. Barzarga, and B. A. Cunha. "Measles: Lessons from an Outbreak." *American Journal of Infection Control* 20 (December 1992): 319–325.

Hazinski, M. F., and R. M. Barkin, eds. *Pediatric Emergency Medicine: Concepts and Clinical Practice.* St. Louis: Mosby, 1992.

Huse, D. M., C. Meissner, M. J. Lacey, and G. Oster. "Childhood Vaccination Against Chickenpox: An Analysis of Benefits and Costs." *Journal of Pediatrics* 124 (June 1994): 869–874.

Klein, J. "Hepatitis B Infection: Maternal—Newborn Evaluation and Management." *Journal of Nursing Staff Development* (July/August 1994): 231–232.

Kulig, K. "Initial Management of Ingestions of Toxic Substances." *New England Journal of Medicine* 326 (June 1992): 1677.

Maloney-Harmon, P. A. "Initial Assessment and Stabilization of the Pediatric Trauma Patient." *Critical Care Medicine* 21 (September 1993): S392–S393.

Reynolds, E. A. "Trauma Scoring and Pediatric Patients: Issues and Controversies." *Journal of Emergency Nursing* 18 (June 1992): 205–209.

Sharts-Hopko, N. C. "Preventing Hepatitis B in Infants." *Maternal Child Nursing* 17 (November/December 1992): 336.

Sumaya, C. V. "Infectious Mono and Epstein-Barr Virus Related Syndromes." In Gillis and Keagan's *Current Pediatric Therapy,* edited by F. D. Burg, J. R. Ingelfinger, and E. R. Wald, 608–609. Philadelphia: W. B. Saunders, 1992.

APPENDIX

RECOMMENDED CHILDHOOD IMMUNIZATION SCHEDULE
UNITED STATES—JANUARY 1995

VACCINE	BIRTH	2 MOS	4 MOS
Hepatitis B[1]	HB-1		
		HB-2	
Diphtheria, tetanus, pertussis[2]		DTP	DTP
H. influenzae type b[3]		Hib	Hib
Polio		OPV	OPV
Measles, mumps, rubella[4]			

VACCINE	6 MOS	12[5] MOS	15 MOS	18 MOS
Hepatitis B[1]	HB-3			
Diphtheria, tetanus, pertussis[2]	DTP	DTP or DTaP at ≥ 15 mos		
H. influenzae type b[3]	Hib	Hib		
Polio	OPV			
Measles, mumps, rubella[4]			MMR	

RECOMMENDED CHILDHOOD IMMUNIZATION SCHEDULE
UNITED STATES—JANUARY 1995 *(CONTINUED)*

VACCINE	4-6 YRS	11-12 YRS	14-16 YRS
Hepatitis B[1]			
Diphtheria, tetanus, pertussis[2]	DTP or DTaP	Td	
H. influenzae type b[3]			
Polio	OPV		
Measles, mumps, rubella[4]		MMR or MMR	

Vaccines are listed under the routinely recommended ages. Shaded bars indicate the range of acceptable ages for vaccination.

[1] Infants born to HBsAg–negative mothers should receive the second dose of hepatits B vaccine between 1 and 4 months of age, provided at least 1 month has elapsed since receipt of the first dose. The third dose is recommeded between 6 and 18 months of age.

Infants born to HBsAg–positive mothers should receive immunoprophy-laxis for hepatits B with 0.5 mL Hepatitis B Immune Globulin (HBIG) within 12 hours of birth, and 0.5 mL of either Merck Sharp & Dohme vaccine (Recombivax HB) or of SmithKline Beecham vaccine (Engerix–B) at a separate site. In these infants, the second dose of vac-cine is recommended at 1 month of age and the third dose at 6 months of age. All pregnant women should be screened for HBsAg in an early prenatal visit.

[2] The fourth dose of DTP may be administered as early as 12 months of age, provided at least 6 months have elapsed since DTP3. Combined DTP-Hib products may be used when these two vaccines are to be administered simultaneously. DTaP (diphtheria and tetanus toxoids

and acellular pertussis vaccine) is licensed for use for the 4th and/or 5th dose of DTP vaccine in children 15 months of age or older and may be preferred for these doses in children in this age-group.

[3]Three *H. influenzae* type b conjugate vaccines are available for use in infants: HbOC (HibTITER) (Lederle Praxis); PRP-T (ActHIB; OmniHIB) (Pasteur Merieux, distributed by SmithKline Beecham; Connaught); and PRP-OMP (PedvaxHIB) (Merck Sharp & Dohme). Children who have received PRP-OMP at 2 and 4 months of age do not require a dose at 6 months of age. After the primary infant Hib conjugate vaccine series is completed, any licensed Hib conjugate vaccine may be used as a booster dose at 12–15 months.

[4]The second dose of MMR vaccine should be administered either at 4–6 years of age or at 11–12 years of age.

[5]Vaccines recommended in the second year of life (12–15 months of age) may be given at either one or two visits.

Approved by the Advisory Committee on Immunization Practices (ACIP), the American Academy of Pediatrics, and the American Academy of Family Physicians (AAFP).

Note that as of the publication date of this book, the varicella vaccine has been approved by the Food and Drug Administration. Consult with health care providers or pharmacists for complete details.

STAGES OF COGNITIVE AND SOCIOEMOTIONAL DEVELOPMENT

Cognitive *

STAGE	LEARNING TO:
Birth to 2 years (Sensorimotor)	• Differentiates self from the world; is achieving some sense of self-identity • Learns through activity, exploration, and manipulation of the environment; motor and sensory skills are forming a basis for subsequent learning • Forms and integrates schemes: knows sucking on a nipple produces milk or shaking a rattle makes noise • Develops object permanence • Uses simple tools
2 to 6/7 years (Preoperational)	• Makes symbolic representations of the world with language, play, and deferred imitation • Not yet capable of sustained, systematic thought • Engages in symbolic play; is less egocentric; uses language and drawing to represent experiences
6/7 to 11 years	• Uses limited logical thought processes: sees relationships and classifies with manipulable, concrete materials • Knows that aspects of articles stay constant despite changes in appearance • Mentally reverses a process of action • Focuses on a number of aspects of a situation at one time • Deduces new relationships from preceding ones • Places things in sequential order and groups things according to common features

STAGES OF COGNITIVE AND SOCIOEMOTIONAL DEVELOPMENT
(CONTINUED)

COGNITIVE *(CONTINUED)*

STAGE	LEARNING TO:
12 through adult (Formal Operations)	• Reasons logically and abstractly • Formulates and tests hypotheses • Thought is not dependent on concrete reality • Explores possibilities • Deals with abstract ideas • Manipulates variables in a scientific situation • Deals with analogies and metaphors • Reflects on own thinking • Works out combinations and permutations

SOCIOEMOTIONAL
Psychosocial †

Birth to 18 months (Trust vs. Mistrust)	• Trusts, or mistrusts, that needs will be met by the world, especially by mother
3 years (Autonomy vs. Shame, Doubt)	• Makes choices and exercises will and self-control
6 years (Initiative vs. Guilt)	• Initiates activities and enjoys accomplishments, acquiring direction and purpose
12 years (Industry vs. Inferiority)	• Has a sense of industry and curiosity; is eager to learn

SOCIOEMOTIONAL
Psychosexual ‡

Birth to 18 months (Oral stage)	• Obtains gratification through stimulation of mouth when biting and sucking

STAGES OF COGNITIVE AND SOCIOEMOTIONAL DEVELOPMENT
(CONTINUED)

SOCIOEMOTIONAL (CONTINUED)

STAGE	LEARNING TO:
3 years (Anal Stage)	• Gets gratification when exercising the anal musculature during elimination or retention
6 years (Phallic [Oedipal] Stage)	• Develops sexual curiosity and is gratified by masturbation • Has sexual fantasies about the opposite-sex parent with accompanying guilt about the fantasies
12 years (Latency Stage)	• Energetically involved in acquiring cultural skills • Sexual urges are submerged
Adolescent (Genital Stage)	• Has adult sexual desires and tries to satisfy them

*Based on Jean Piaget.
†Based on Erik Erikson.
‡Based on Sigmund Freud.
Source: Behrman and Kliegman: Nelson's Essentials of Pediatrics, 1990.

INDEX

A

ABCs as assessment component, 3
Acne, 150
  documentation for, 152
  impaired skin integrity and, 151
  patient teaching for, 152
Acute otitis externa
  documentation for, 48
  pain and, 47-48
  patient teaching for, 48
Acute otitis media, 48
  documentation for, 50
  pain and, 49-50
  patient teaching for, 50
Acute renal failure, 117
  documentation for, 119
  fluid volume excess and, 117-119
  patient teaching for, 119
Adenoidectomy, 37
Adenoiditis, 37
Adolescent
  developmental characteristics of, 23
  sexual development concerns and,
    99-102
Airway, assessing, 3, 22, 29
Aortic stenosis, 74. See also Congenital
  heart disease.
Appendicitis, 91
  documentation for, 93
  high risk for fluid volume deficit and,
    92-93
  pain and, 91-92
  patient teaching for, 93
Arrhythmias, 64
  decreased cardiac output and, 65-66,
    67-68
  documentation for, 70
  inadequate tissue perfusion and, 69-70
  patient teaching for, 70
Asthma, 59
  documentation for, 61
  impaired gas exchange and, 59-61
  ineffective airway clearance and, 59-61
  patient teaching for, 61
Asystole, 68
Atrial septal defect, 72-73. See also
  Congenital heart disease.
Auscultation, blood pressure measurement and, 26
Axillary temperature, 27, 28

B

Bedwetting. See Enuresis.
Blood pressure
  abnormal, nursing interventions for,
    10-11
  measuring, 26-27
Bradyarrhythmia, 64-66
Breathing, assessing, 3, 22, 29
Burns
  classifying, 152-153
  documentation for, 157
  high risk for infection and, 156-157
  impaired skin integrity and, 154-155
  pain and, 155-156
  patient teaching for, 157

C

Cardiovascular disorders, nursing diag-
  noses for, 65-81
Chickenpox, 168
  documentation for, 170
  knowledge deficit and, 169
  patient teaching for, 170
Child abuse, types of, 134
Childhood infections, 168-181
Chlamydial infection, 103. See also
  Sexually transmitted diseases.
Circulation, assessing, 3, 22, 29
Coarctation of the aorta, 75. See also
  Congenital heart disease.
Cognitive development, stages
  of, 204-205
Colic, nursing research and, 94
Collapse rhythms, 68-70
Communication
  as assessment component, 4-5
  as nursing intervention, 6-8
Congenital heart disease, 71-72
  documentation for, 78-79
  ineffective family coping and, 77-78
  patient teaching for, 78
  types of, 72-76
Congenital hip dysplasia, 128
  documentation for, 130
  knowledge deficit and, 129-130
  patient teaching for, 130
Congestive heart failure, 79
  decreased cardiac output and, 79-80

documentation for, 81
ineffective breathing pattern and, 80-81
nursing research and, 82
patient teaching for, 81
Constipation, 89
documentation for, 91
interventions for, 89-90
patient teaching for, 90-91
Croup, 55
anxiety and, 57-58
documentation for, 58
ineffective airway clearance and, 55-57
patient teaching for, 58

Defibrillation, 70-71
Dehydration, signs of, 83
Developmental functioning, assessing, 33
Development assessment considerations, 23
Diaper dermatitis, 147
Doppler blood pressure measurement, 26

Eczema, 148
Enuresis, 119
documentation for, 121
knowledge deficit and, 120-121
patient teaching for, 121
Epiglottiditis, 52
documentation for, 55
impaired gas exchange and, 52-54
ineffective airway clearance and, 52-54
patient teaching for, 55
Epistaxis, 43
anxiety and, 46
documentation for, 47
high risk for fluid volume deficit and, 44-45
patient teaching for, 46
Epstein-Barr virus infection, 178
documentation for, 179
pain and, 178-179
patient teaching for, 179

Fetal circulation, anatomical changes in, 76
Fever, 159-167
assessing child with, 161
causes of, 159-160
documentation for, 167
effects of, 160-161

fluid volume deficit and, 163-164
hyperthermia and, 161-163
incidence of, 159
knowledge deficit and, 165-166
managing, 159
nursing research and, 167
patient teaching for, 166
as sign, 159
Fractures
documentation for, 128
impaired physical mobility and, 124-127
pain and, 123-124
patient teaching for, 128
types of, 122

Gastroenteritis, 83
altered nutrition (less than body requirements) and, 85-86
diarrhea and, 87
documentation for, 89
fluid volume deficit and, 84-85
patient teaching for, 88-89
Gastrointestinal disorders, nursing diagnoses for, 84-87
Genital herpes, 104. *See also* Sexually transmitted diseases.
Gonorrhea, 102. *See also* Sexually transmitted diseases.
Growth assessment considerations, 23

Head and neck assessment considerations, 22
Head and neck infections, 37-43
decreased cardiac output and, 41-42
documentation for, 43
high risk for infection and, 39
ineffective airway clearance and, 38-39, 40-41
pain and, 40, 42
patient teaching for, 43
Head circumference, measuring, 29
Head injuries, 137
documentation for, 139-140
high risk for injury and, 137-139
patient teaching for, 139
Head lice, 149
Health history, 13-21
guidelines for collecting, 13-14
key components of, 13
subject areas for, 14-21
Height, measuring, 28, 29

Hepatitis, 170
  altered nutrition (less than body
    requirements) and, 170-171
  documentation for, 172
  patient teaching for, 171
Herpes simplex, 149
Human immunodeficiency virus infec-
    tion, 105. *See also* Sexually transmit-
    ted diseases.
Human papillomavirus, 104. *See also*
    Sexually transmitted diseases.
Hypertension, nursing interventions for,
    10
Hypotension, nursing interventions for,
    10-11
Hypoxia, signs and symptoms of, 24

I

Immunization schedule, 201-203
Impetigo, 149
Infant
  developmental characteristics of, 23
  sexual development concerns and,
    95-96
Intracranial pressure, increased, 140
  documentation for, 143
  high risk for injury and, 140-141
  ineffective breathing pattern and, 142
  patient teaching for, 143

L

Laryngotracheobronchitis. *See* Croup.
Level of consciousness, evaluating, 31-32

M

Measles, 172
  documentation for, 173
  pain and, 172-173
  patient teaching for, 173
Meningitis, 145
  documentation for, 146
  high risk for infection and, 145-146
  patient teaching for, 146
Mumps, 173
  documentation for, 175
  pain and, 174
  patient teaching for, 174
Musculoskeletal disorders, nursing diag-
    noses for, 123-127

N

Neglect, 134
Nephrotic syndrome, 115

  documentation for, 117
  fluid volume excess and, 115-116
  high risk for infection and, 116
  patient teaching for, 117
Neurologic problems, nursing diagnoses
    for, 137-146
Neurologic status, assessing, 3, 30-32
Nosebleed. *See* Epistaxis.
Nursing interventions, 6-12

O

Observation as assessment component,
    2-3
Oral temperature, 27, 28

P

Pain assessment, 32
Pain management, nursing interventions
    for, 11-12
Palpation, blood pressure measurement
    and, 26
Patent ductus arteriosus, 74. *See also*
    Congenital heart disease.
Pediculosis capitis, 149
Pelvic inflammatory disease, 103. *See also*
    Sexually transmitted diseases.
Pertussis. *See* Whooping cough.
Physical assessment, 22-36
  components of, 1-5
Poisoning, 182-187
  documentation for, 187
  high risk for injury and, 184-186
  patient teaching for, 186-187
  signs and symptoms of, 182-184
Preschooler
  developmental characteristics of, 23
  sexual development concerns and,
    96-98
Pulmonary stenosis, 74. *See also*
    Congenital heart disease.
Pulse, abnormal, nursing interventions
    for, 10
Pulse rate, assessing, 25-26
Pupil size, variation of, in altered con-
    sciousness, 30

R

Rape. *See* Sexual assault.
Rash, 147
  documentation for, 150
  patient teaching for, 150

Rectal temperature, 27, 28
Reproductive system, knowledge deficit related to, 95-102
Respiratory disorders, nursing diagnoses for, 51-63
Respiratory distress
  factors leading to, 51
  nursing interventions for, 9
  signs of, 24
Respiratory rate, assessing, 24
Respiratory syncytial virus, 61-62
  documentation for, 63
  impaired gas exchange and, 62-63
  ineffective airway clearance and, 62-63
  nursing research and, 63
  patient teaching for, 63
Review of systems, 17-21, 37-157
Rheumatic fever, 176
Ringworm, 150
Roseola, 150
Rubella, 175
  documentation for, 176
  knowledge deficit and, 175-176
  patient teaching for, 176
Rubeola. *See* Measles.

S

Scabies, 149
Scarlatina, 176
Scarlet fever, 176
School-age child
  developmental characteristics of, 23
  sexual development concerns and, 98-99
Scoliosis, 130
  documentation for, 133
  ineffective individual coping, 132-133
  noncompliance and, 132-133
  patient teaching for, 133
  types of, 131
Seborrhea, 148
Secondary assessment, 33-36
Sexual assault, 110
  documentation for, 112
  high risk for injury and, 111
  patient teaching for, 112
Sexually transmitted diseases, 102
  documentation for, 108
  knowledge deficit and, 105-107
  patient teaching for, 107
  types of, 102-105
Shock, 196
  altered tissue perfusion and, 196-197
  documentation for, 199

high risk for infection and, 197-198
  patient teaching for, 199
Sinus tachycardia, 66
Skeletal trauma from abuse, 134
  documentation for, 136
  high risk for injury and, 135-136
  patient teaching for, 136
Skin, function of, 147
Skin problems, types of, 147-150
Socioemotional development, stages of, 205-206
Status epilepticus, 143-144
  altered cerebral tissue perfusion and, 144
  patient teaching for, 145
Strep throat, 176
  documentation for, 178
  pain and, 177
  patient teaching for, 177
Supraventricular tachycardia, 66
Swimmer's ear. *See* Acute otitis externa.
Synchronized cardioversion, 70-71
Syphilis, 103. *See also* Sexually transmitted diseases.

T

Tachyarrhythmia, 66-68
Teenage pregnancy
  altered health maintenance management and, 108-109
  complications of, 108
  documentation for, 110
  incidence of, 108
  patient teaching for, 110
Temperature, measuring, 27-28
Tetralogy of Fallot, 75. *See also* Congenital heart disease.
Thermoregulation assessment considerations, 23
Tinea corporis, 150
Toddler
  developmental characteristics of, 23
  sexual development concerns and, 95-96
Tonsillar anatomy, 38
Tonsillectomy, 37
Tonsillitis, 37
Toxic substances, 182-184
Transcultural considerations, assessment and, 5
Transposition of the great arteries, 76. *See also* Congenital heart disease.
Trauma
  documentation for, 195
  high risk for injury and, 190-195

incidence of, 188
patient teaching for, 195
types of, 188-190
Trichomoniasis, 104. *See also* Sexually
transmitted diseases.
Tympanic temperature, 27-28, 167

U

Ultrasonographic blood pressure measurement, 26
Urinary tract infection, 113
documentation for, 114
high risk for infection and, 113-114
patient teaching for, 114

V

Ventricular fibrillation, 68
Ventricular septal defect, 73. *See also*
Congenital heart disease.
Vital signs, assessing, 3, 8-9, 22, 23-29

W

Weight, measuring, 28, 29
Whooping cough, 179
documentation for, 181
ineffective breathing pattern and, 180
nursing research and, 181
patient teaching for, 180

ORDER OTHER TITLES IN THIS SERIES!

INSTANT NURSING ASSESSMENT:

▲ Cardiovascular	0-8273-7102-0
▲ Respiratory	0-8273-7099-7
▲ Neurologic	0-8273-7103-9
▲ Women's Health	0-8273-7100-4
▲ Gerontologic	0-8273-7101-2
▲ Mental Health	0-8273-7104-7
▲ Pediatric	0-8273-7098-9

RAPID NURSING INTERVENTIONS

▲ Cardiovascular	0-8273-7105-5
▲ Respiratory	0-8273-7095-4
▲ Neurologic	0-8273-7093-8
▲ Women's Health	0-8273-7092-X
▲ Gerontologic	0-8273-7094-6
▲ Mental Health	0-8273-7096-2
▲ Pediatric	0-8273-7097-0

- (cut here) -

EXPERIENCE AT YOUR FINGERTIPS!

QTY.	TITLE / ISBN	PRICE	TOTAL
		19.95	
		19.95	
		19.95	
		19.95	
		19.95	
		19.95	
		SUBTOTAL	
		STATE OR LOCAL TAXES	
		TOTAL	

Payment Information
☐ A Check is Enclosed
☐ Charge my ☐ VISA ☐ Mastercard CARD #_____

MAIL OR FAX COMPLETED FORM TO:
Delmar Publishers • P.O. Box 15015 • Albany, NY 12212-5015

NAME_____

SCHOOL/INSTITUTION _____

STREET ADDRESS_____

CITY/STATE/ZIP _____

HOME PHONE_____

OFFICE PHONE_____

IN A HURRY TO ORDER? FAX: 1-518-464-0301
OR CALL TOLL-FREE 1-800-347-7707